The Essential Guide to Coding Audits

JustCoding

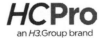

The Essential Guide to Coding Audits is published by HCPro, an H3.Group division of Simplify Compliance, LLC.

Download this book's appendix at *www.hcpro.com/downloads/12651*

ISBN: 978-1-68308-710-6

HCPro provides information resources for the healthcare industry.

HCPro is not affiliated in any way with The Joint Commission, which owns the JCAHO and Joint Commission trademarks.

Rose T. Dunn, MBA, RHIA, CPA/CGMA, FACHE, FHFMA, CHPS, Author
William L. Malm, ND, RN, CRCR, CMAS, Contributor
Amanda Norris, Editor
Andrea Kraynak, Product Manager
Erin Callahan, Vice President, Product Development and Content Strategy
Matt Sharpe, Production Supervisor
Vincent Skyers, Design Services Director
Dawn Stratchko, Layout/Graphic Design
Jason Gregory, Cover Designer

Advice given is general. Readers should consult professional counsel for specific legal, ethical, or clinical questions.

Arrangements can be made for quantity discounts. For more information, contact:

HCPro
35 Village Road, Suite 200
Middleton, MA 01949
Telephone: 800-650-6787 or 781-639-1872
Fax: 800-785-9212
Email: *customerservice@hcpro.com*

Visit HCPro online at www.hcpro.com and www.hcmarketplace.com

Contents

Chapter 5: Audit Focus and the Approach of Insurers............73

About the Authors

Rose T. Dunn, MBA, RHIA, CPA/CGMA, FACHE, FHFMA, CHPS is a past president of the American Health Information Management Association (AHIMA) and recipient of its 1997 Distinguished Member and 2008 Legacy awards. In 2011, Dunn served as the interim chief executive officer of AHIMA and received a Distinguished Service Award from the board of directors. Dunn is the chief operating officer of First Class Solutions, Inc., a health information management (HIM) consulting firm in St. Louis, Missouri. Dunn began her career as director of medical records at Barnes Hospital, which at that time was a 1,200-bed teaching hospital in St. Louis. It is now the flagship hospital of the BJC HealthCare system. Early in her career at Barnes, she became vice president and was responsible for more than 1,600 employees and new business development. She later joined Metropolitan Life Insurance Company, where she served as assistant vice president in MetLife's HMO subsidiary. She also served as chief financial officer of a dual-hospital system in Illinois and was heavily involved in its successful bond application.

Her consulting firm, First Class Solutions, Inc., focuses primarily on HIM-related services, including coding support, coding audits, and operations improvement. Dunn assists clients with their operational, revenue cycle, compliance, and strategic planning needs. Dunn is active in several professional associations, including the American Institute of Certified Public Accountants, American College of

Healthcare Executives (ACHE), Healthcare Financial Management Association (HFMA), National Association of Healthcare Revenue Integrity (NAHRI), and AHIMA. She holds fellowship status in ACHE, AHIMA, and HFMA and is certified by AHIMA in healthcare privacy and security.

Dunn's previously published books include *JustCoding's Practical Guide to Coding Management, Coder Productivity: Tapping Your Team's Talents to Improve Quality,* and *Reduce Accounts Receivable and More with Less: Best Practices for HIM Directors,* first and second editions, published by HCPro. She is the coauthor of *The Practical Guide to Release of Information* and *The Practical Guide to Release of Information: ROI in a HITECH World,* both also published by HCPro. She is the coauthor of *Finance Principles for the Health Information Manager,* published by First Class Solutions, Inc., and *Dunn and Haimann's Healthcare Management,* 10th edition, published by Health Administration Press. Dunn is also the author of the NAHRI publication *The Revenue Integrity Manager's Guidebook.*

Dunn is the author of more than 225 articles and is a frequent speaker on various management, regulatory, compliance, coding, and healthcare topics.

Contributor: William L. Malm, ND, RN, CRCR, CMAS, is a managing director at Health Revenue Integrity Services. Malm wrote Chapter 5, "Audit Focus and the Approach of Insurers," of this book. He is a nationally recognized author and speaker on topics such as healthcare compliance, chargemasters, and CMS recovery audits. Malm brings more than 25 years of experience with a combination of clinical and financial healthcare knowledge that encompasses all aspects of revenue integrity. He also serves as the secretary/treasurer for the Certification Council of Medical Auditors. He has extensive experience with all postpayment audits, having previously worked as a systems compliance officer at a large for-profit healthcare system. Malm also cohosts Appeal Academy's "Finally Friday" discussions.

Acknowledgments

This book is dedicated to the talented coding professionals at First Class Solutions, Inc., with whom I have had the honor to work for 30 years. Thank you for your commitment to our clients you serve and your determination to ensure data integrity through compliant and high-quality coding.

No book is ever the product of one person's efforts. Many individuals contributed to its development, editing, formatting, and publication. I was fortunate to have some of the best working with me on this edition. Editor Amanda Norris thoroughly reviewed the manuscript and offered many valuable suggestions while keeping the production running smoothly. Jason Gregory, cover designer, and Dawn Stratchko, graphic artist, designed the book's interior, respectively. Amanda Donaldson served as the proofreader. To them and those other individuals working behind the scenes, thank you.

Rose T. Dunn

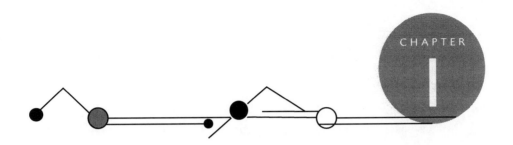

Introduction to Coding Audits

CHAPTER OBJECTIVES

- Overview of why the practice of auditing coding began
- Review of the significant regulatory activities assessing the accuracy of coding
- Discuss the reasons coding professionals should comply with the *Standards of Ethical Coding*
- Discuss the purpose of a corporate integrity agreement
- Recognize professional and health-related association guidance of ethical coding practice

What Is a Coding Audit?

While I prefer the use of the term "coding review," the industry commonly uses the term "coding audit" as the practice of reviewing the accuracy of code assignment. These audits are done based on the documentation in the patient's record at the time of the review, which is then compared against the codes that were reported on that claim.

The review should be more encompassing than solely looking at the accuracy of the codes assigned.

The reviews should be used to identify:

- Other conditions that are documented and not coded (coding omissions). These additional conditions may lead to a comorbidity/complication (CC) or major CC (MCC), which increases the degree of morbidity or risk of mortality for the patient, thus painting a picture of the patient's severity of illness. This could also contribute to an additional hierarchical condition category or ambulatory payment classification, which may increase reimbursement.

- Opportunities to seek further clarity and specificity for those conditions that were documented and coded with limited specificity or unspecified or conditions implied based on tests performed, medications administered, and other clinical indications, but were not documented by the physicians. These are cases in which physician queries may have enhanced the coding process but were not issued.

- Documentation issues for one or more providers or documentation issues fostered by the electronic health record or templates/forms designed for provider use.

- Charges that appear on the claim but are not supported by the documentation in the record.

Reasons for Coding Scrutiny

In an industry that is under the microscope by multiple entities, coding is at the forefront of those activities being scrutinized and has been for years. When the United States Medicare inpatient reimbursement methodology converted from a retrospective cost-based approach in the mid-1980s to a prospective reimbursement system utilizing diagnosis-related groups (DRG), the need for federal intervention for assessing the accuracy of coding by hospitals arose.

Understandingly so, the government needed to do its due diligence to ensure it was not overpaying for services. Since commercial insurers routinely mirror the

The Essential Guide to Coding Audits

reimbursement approaches of the Centers for Medicare & Medicaid Services (CMS), it was not surprising to see major carriers adopt the DRG payment approach for inpatient stays.

During the early years of the inpatient prospective payment system (IPPS), the availability of technologies to guide coders on DRG assignment, such as an encoder, was absent or limited. The use of manual DRG trees was the primary tool used by coders, which left opportunity for error. Over time, the prospective payment approach has been applied to the provider and ambulatory healthcare markets, and technologies have advanced to facilitate the assignment of codes and their prospective payment categories.

For many professional providers, the use of the evaluation and management (E/M) code has driven their reimbursement. There are two approaches to E/M code assignment, the 1995 and 1997 Documentation Guidelines for Evaluation and Management Services, both of which are accepted by CMS. A provider does not need to choose one set of guidelines or the other when determining which E/M code to assign for his or her practice. A provider may use the 1995 criteria on one encounter and use the 1997 criteria on another. Historically, there was a limitation that the provider could not blend both for a single encounter, but that changed in 2013 with CMS' decision to allow some limited blending of the criteria for the history of present illness: "… beginning for services performed on or after September 10, 2013, physicians may use the 1997 documentation guidelines for an extended history of present illness along with other elements from the 1995 guidelines to document an evaluation and management service" (CMS, n.d.).

There are differences between the two criteria sets. Due to the structural differences of the guidelines, specialists may prefer the 1997 criteria, which focus on specific body systems that are of interest by specialists and also include the counseling time approach, while primary care providers (PCP) may prefer the 1995 criteria, which capture the broad evaluation often performed by PCPs. External auditors will pay close attention to the provider's billing patterns and coding practices to determine whether there are variations that warrant a closer look at the actual documentation. Figure 1.1 is from the Medicare contractor Palmetto GBA and provides a comparison of the two guidelines (Palmetto GBA, 2016).

FIGURE 1.1 DIFFERENCES BETWEEN THE 1995 AND 1997 E/M DOCUMENTATION GUIDELINES

	1995	*1997*
E/M Components		
History of the present illness	No difference*	No difference*
Review of systems	No difference	No difference
History		
Past, family, and social	No difference	No difference
Examination**	Body areas, body systems, or complete single organ system (e.g., cardiovascular, eyes, psychiatric, etc.)	General multisystem or single organ system (e.g., cardiovascular, eyes, psychiatric, etc.)
Decision-making	No difference	No difference

* An extended history of present illness may consist of the status of three chronic/inactive conditions for either set of guidelines (1995 or 1997) for services performed on or after September 10, 2013.

** A detailed exam involves 6 or 7 body areas or organ systems; an expanded problem-focused exam involves 2–5 body areas or organ systems effective July 1, 2017.

Adapted source: Palmetto GBA, 2016.

Note: Additional information to assist in understanding the differences between the two guidelines is available from HCPro at hcpro.com/HIM-242234-8160/Understand-how-to-apply-the-1995-and-1997-Documentation-Guidelines-for-EM-Services.html or E/M University at http://emuniversity.com/FAQ/EMFAQ3.html.

Following the Guidelines

All providers (facilities and professionals) should abide by the *ICD-10-CM* and *ICD-10-PCS Official Guidelines for Coding and Reporting* published by CMS. Professionals and outpatient facilities use the diagnosis portion of the coding guidelines, the American Medical Association's *CPT® Assistant*, and information contained in the CPT-4® book for their procedural coding. Inpatient facilities use the coding guidelines and guidance contained in the American Hospital Association's *Coding Clinic* for both diagnosis and procedural coding.

Auditing professionals should be well versed in the guidance provided by these primary sources and know how to access the coding rules discussed in the National Correct Coding Initiative (NCCI) and the *Medicare Claims Processing Manual*. Regardless of the coding environment (facility or professional practice), there remains opportunity for error, either unintentional or intentional. Thus, there is a need for auditing all coding activities.

Regulatory Concerns

Since most services today are provided for patients with either governmental or private insurance, the interest in accurate coding is highest among the payers, and there are many governmental agencies that may conduct audits. However, all governmental auditors have a common goal: to protect governmental funds from being misused. Often, they are categorized under the heading of "fraud and abuse."

Fraud and abuse

Fraud and abuse are extensively covered by the Office of Inspector General (OIG) and includes programs such as the Civil False Claims Act, Comprehensive Error Rate Testing, and the NCCI (Dunn, 2016).

The Civil False Claims Act

The Civil False Claims Act has a long history, having been implemented during the Civil War. It states that (CMS, 2007):

> *Any person who (1) **knowingly** presents, or causes to be presented, to … the United States Government … a false or fraudulent claim for payment or approval; (2) **knowingly** makes, uses, or causes to be made or used, a false record or statement to get a false or fraudulent claim paid or approved by the Government; (3) conspires to defraud the Government by getting a false or fraudulent claim paid or approved by the Government; … or (7) **knowingly** makes, uses, or causes to be made or used, a false record or statement to conceal, avoid, or decrease an obligation to pay or transmit money or property to the Government … is liable to the United States Government for a civil penalty of not less than $5,000 and not more than $10,000, plus 3 times the amount of damages which the Government sustains because of the act of that person …*
>
> *(b) For purposes of this section, the terms "knowing" and "knowingly" mean that a person, with respect to information (1) has actual knowledge of the information; (2) acts in deliberate ignorance of the truth or falsity of the information; or (3) acts in reckless disregard of the truth or falsity of the information, and no proof of specific intent to defraud is required.*

NCCI

The NCCI was developed by CMS to promote national correct coding methodologies and to control improper coding leading to inappropriate payment in Part B claims (CMS, 2018). CMS developed its coding policies based on coding conventions defined in the American Medical Association's *CPT Manual*, national and local policies and edits, coding guidelines developed by national societies, analysis of standard medical and surgical practices, and a review of current coding practices. CMS annually updates the *NCCI Coding Policy Manual for Medicare Services (Coding Policy Manual)*. The *Coding Policy Manual* should be utilized by carriers and fiscal intermediaries (FI) as a general reference tool that explains the rationale for NCCI edits (Dunn, 2016).

Carriers implemented NCCI procedure-to-procedure (PTP) edits within their claim processing systems for dates of service on or after January 1, 1996, and began implementing medically unlikely edits (MUE) on January 1, 2007.

A corresponding set of PTP edits is incorporated into the outpatient code editor for OPPS and therapy providers (Part B skilled nursing facilities, comprehensive outpatient rehabilitation facilities, outpatient physical therapy and speech-language pathology providers, and certain claims for home health agency billing).

The purpose of the NCCI PTP edits is to prevent improper payment when incorrect code combinations are reported. The NCCI contains one table of edits for physicians/practitioners and one table of edits for outpatient hospital services. The purpose of the NCCI MUE program is to prevent improper payments when services are reported with incorrect units of service.

Within the organization's billing system and/or encoding system, edits will be incorporated to alert the coder of some or all of the NCCI rule edits. When the system allows an option to "turn off" the edits from view, the coding professional is not afforded the guidance the NCCI edits provide and therefore may apply a code to a claim that will result in a rejection or denial. Ensuring the edits are in a viewable mode is the ideal way to ensure compliance with these national coding rules.

OIG Work Plan

The OIG publishes a *Work Plan* annually and semiannually. The OIG *Work Plan* sets forth various projects to be addressed during the fiscal year by the Office of Audit Services, Office of Evaluation and Inspections, Office of Investigations, and Office of Counsel to the Inspector General.

The *Work Plan* includes projects planned in each of the department's major entities, including CMS, the public health agencies, the Administrations for Children and Families, and Administration on Aging. Information is also provided on projects related to issues that cut across departmental programs, including state and local government use of federal funds, as well as the functional areas of the Office of the Secretary of Health & Human Services (HHS) (OIG, n.d.a.).

While most OIG activities that relate to coding appear in the Medicare & Medicaid Services section of the *Work Plan,* it is worthwhile to peruse the other sections for pertinent items that affect your organization. The 2017 *Work Plan*, as well as previous plans, are available at *oig.hhs.gov/reports-and-publications/archives/workplan/index.asp#2017.*

Coding ethics

So, what does all this mean for coding professionals? Because coding professionals supply many of the codes that appear on the claim and drive the reimbursement for facility and professional providers, they are contributing to the claim that is submitted to the government. If the coding professional knowingly supplies a code that will increase the reimbursement and knowingly recognizes that the documentation in the patient record does not support the code(s), then that claim could be considered "false" and subject to the civil penalties noted earlier. Of course, the coder could be subject to disciplinary actions by the employer and possibly civil action. If the coding professional is running a billing service on behalf of several providers, the billing service could be subject to the penalties and a possible jail sentence.

Coding professionals are encouraged to follow ethical coding practices regardless of whether there is a governmental or private payer involved. AHIMA's *Standards of Ethical Coding* are based on AHIMA's *Code of Ethics*. Both sets of principles reflect expectation of professional conduct for coding professionals involved in diagnostic and/or procedural coding or other health record data abstraction. AHIMA's standards are summarized in 11 key ethical coding principles that appear in Figure 1.2. Additional content regarding the standards is available on the AHIMA website.

FIGURE 1.2

AHIMA's 2016 Standards of Ethical Coding
1. Apply accurate, complete, and consistent coding practices that yield quality data.
2. Gather and report all data required for internal and external reporting, in accordance with applicable requirements and data set definitions
3. Assign and report, in any format, only the codes and data that are clearly and consistently supported by health record documentation in accordance with applicable code set and abstraction conventions and requirements.
4. Query and/or consult as needed with the provider for clarification and additional documentation prior to final code assignment in accordance with acceptable healthcare industry practices.
5. Refuse to participate in, support, or change reported data and/or narrative titles, billing data, clinical documentation practices, or any coding-related activities intended to skew or misrepresent data and their meaning that do not comply with requirements.
6. Facilitate, advocate, and collaborate with healthcare professionals in the pursuit of accurate, complete, and reliable coded data and in situations that support ethical coding practices.
7. Advance coding knowledge and practice through continuing education, including but not limited to meeting continuing education requirements.
8. Maintain the confidentiality of protected health information in accordance with the Code of Ethics.
9. Refuse to participate in the development of coding and coding-related technology that is not designed in accordance with requirements.
10. Demonstrate behavior that reflects integrity, shows a commitment to ethical and legal coding practices, and fosters trust in professional activities.
11. Refuse to participate in and/or conceal unethical coding, data abstraction, query practices, or any inappropriate activities related to coding and address any perceived unethical coding-related practices.

Source: Bryant, G. H. 2017. "AHIMA's Revised Standards of Ethical Coding Available." Retrieved from http://bok.ahima.org/doc?oid=302300#.WkQC798m7J4. Reprinted with permission from AHIMA.

We encourage our coding team to strive for coding quality and data integrity. Changing a single digit or character of the code to achieve a CC or MCC that yields greater reimbursement for an organization may be tempting. However, such an action could be fraudulent because it implies that the patient record contains sufficient documentation to support the codes that were assigned. Knowingly doing so may create patterns that suggest to oversight entities that an organization engages in questionable practices. These inappropriate practices are often caught when claims data trending analyses are performed.

Upon observation of such practices, oversight and payer entities may request copies of patient records to have their auditors review. Facilities (or providers) may incur financial and licensure penalties, negative publicity, and continuing oversight by government agencies if fraudulent activity is confirmed. As part of the continuing oversight, some facilities (or providers) may be required to submit for approval and monitoring, also known as a corporate integrity agreement (CIA). If the fraudulent activity is determined to be intentional by one or more coders, the coders may lose their certifications and credentials.

Corporate Integrity Agreements

According to Joan Hogarth and Roselyn Tyson of the American Health Lawyers Association, a CIA is an enforcement tool used by the OIG, within the HHS, to improve the quality of healthcare and to promote compliance to healthcare regulations. Similarly, the term integrity agreement is used for smaller healthcare providers such as physicians (AHLA, n.d.).

The CIA is usually entered into contemporaneously with a civil settlement between the government and a healthcare provider (individual and entity) who has been the subject of investigations arising under the False Claims Act as amended in 1986 or who has been found guilty in acts of defrauding Medicare, Medicaid, or any other federal healthcare programs. According to the OIG's website, "a provider or entity consents to these obligations as part of the civil settlement and in exchange for the OIG's agreement not to seek an exclusion of that healthcare provider or entity from participation in Medicare, Medicaid, and other Federal healthcare programs" (OIG, n.d.b.).

CIAs are negotiated and monitored through the Office of Counsel to the Inspector General. They are detailed agreements that are constructed to mirror the Federal Sentencing Guidelines of 1995 while remaining individualized to reflect the scope and size of the healthcare provider and the specific charges that gave rise to that particular CIA.

A CIA allows a provider who has engaged in fraudulent conduct to continue participating in federal healthcare programs. The average time period for a CIA is typically five years. If the healthcare provider breaches the CIA, the OIG reserves the right to impose additional sanctions, including stipulated penalties and permissive exclusion pursuant to its authority under 42 U.S.C.1320a-7(b)(7) (AHLA, n.d.).

Seeking Guidance to Support Coding Quality and Integrity

Coders have an obligation to ensure that coding accurately reflects the services provided. The integrity of the data that coders collect provides valuable information for planning, performance improvement activities, outcome-related reimbursement incentives, epidemiological studies, research, and, of course, claim reimbursement.

For coding integrity, however, coding professionals must abide by their professional association code of ethical conduct. Some of these professional associations include:

- AAPC: Formerly American Academy of Professional Coders, the AAPC is not a member of the Cooperating Parties but is one of the certification entities for coding professionals. Its focus includes providing education, resource materials and publications, and audit software. AAPC provides a forum for coding discussions and several free coding and billing solutions. AAPC has been the forerunner in certifying coding professionals in the requirements of coding for risk adjustment reimbursement.

- American Health Information Management Association (AHIMA): AHIMA is a member of the Cooperating Parties and one of the credentialing and certification entities for coding professionals. Its focus includes:

  – Providing coding education

  – Identifying issues requiring further clarification in the *ICD-10-CM/PCS Official Guidelines for Coding and Reporting* and *Coding Clinic* rules

  – Offering solutions to coding guideline inconsistencies, presenting new conditions and procedure that may require unique codes, and identifying complex coding issues identified by its staff, volunteers, and members for consideration by the Cooperating Parties

- American Hospital Association (AHA): The AHA is a member of the Cooperating Parties. It also publishes *Coding Clinic,* a quarterly newsletter that supplements the *Official ICD-10-CM/PCS Guidelines for Coding and Reporting,* by providing specific examples and clarifying complex and confusing topics. Encoder applications often incorporate *Coding Clinic* to provide coders access to its guidance in real time. These applications trigger alerts as coders assign a code for which *Coding Clinic* rules and/ or official ICD-10-CM and PCS guidelines advice are available. *Coding Clinic* also is available for HCPCS.

- Coding managers may submit coding questions related to ICD-10-CM and PCS codes for inpatient scenarios to the AHA central office at *www. ahacentraloffice.org/codes/ICD10.shtml.*

- However, if the question or recommendation is related to:
  - The ICD-10-CM Index or Tabular List problems or conflicting instructions, questions should be sent to:

    Donna Pickett, RHIA, Medical Classification Administrator
    Office of Planning and Extramural Programs, National Center for
    Health Statistics, Centers for Disease Control
    3311 Toledo Road, Hyattsville, MD 20782

  - The ICD-10-PCS Index entries, ICD-10-PCS device definitions, *ICD-10-PCS Reference Manual*, or the General Equivalence Mappings, questions should be sent to:

    Patricia Brooks, RHIA, Technical Advisor
    CMS, Division of Acute Care, Mail Stop C4-08-06
    7500 Security Boulevard, Baltimore, MD 21244-1850

- American Medical Association (AMA): The AMA is not a member of the Cooperating Parties, but it owns and publishes the CPT coding system used in outpatient coding and physician offices. Because the AMA controls CPT, it also provides guidance for its coding system via its publication, *CPT Assistant*. With respect to ICD-10-CM, coding practices differ between inpatient and outpatient settings. Hospitals will use CPT to code outpatient procedures and ICD-10-PCS for coding its inpatient procedures. Physicians will use CPT for all of the services they performed, regardless of whether they serve as an inpatient or outpatient. All healthcare providers use ICD-10-CM for coding diagnoses. Recognizing the differences is important for coding professionals. Using both systems correctly requires a thorough understanding of the rules that apply to each.

- CMS: CMS is one of many agencies of the HHS. It participates in coding oversight and establishes rules for billing health services and defines which services Medicare will cover. CMS' website (*www.cms.gov*) is comprehensive, complex, and a vital resource for coding managers. Its site facilitates access to information, including but not limited to:

- Educational materials for coders and clinicians (e.g., modifier -59 article)

- Medical necessity guidance, including conditions that qualify for certain tests (i.e., Medicare Coverage Database)

- Program transmittals that clarify documentation and billing requirements (e.g., documentation guidelines for E/M)

- Medicare billing guidelines

• Cooperating Parties: The Cooperating Parties include the AHA, AHIMA, CMS, and National Center for Health Statistics. This group developed and approved the *ICD-10-CM* and *PCS Official Guidelines for Coding and Reporting.* These guidelines, which appear near the beginning of most published ICD-10-CM or ICD-10-PCS manuals, are extensive. New conditions and procedures necessitate the Cooperating Parties' routine review and modification of these manuals. Updates are published no less often than quarterly.

In addition to these national entities, there are opportunities for educational programming through local and regional professional associations, online resources through a number of qualified vendors, and reference materials published by reputable organizations.

There is an abundance of resources available for coding leadership to use to help the coding team produce high-quality data that is accurate, comprehensive, and credible. It is leadership's responsibility to ensure the team has the resources it needs and to provide resources when it's apparent that certain concepts have not been understood based on audit findings and denials.

Conducting routine audits using internal staff or external consultants will assist an organization in reinforcing the ethical coding standards as well as proactively identifying patterns, weaknesses, and errors that can be mitigated through additional education or reassignment of personnel who are unable to achieve the level of coding quality expected by the organization.

Summary

Ever since the 1983 implementation of the IPPS for hospitals and its successor PPS programs, both governmental and commercial payers have monitored the accuracy of the codes submitted by providers. Since codes drive the reimbursement, this practice is appropriate. Therefore, prospective coding auditing by the healthcare organization or healthcare professional is equally appropriate to address reasons for coding errors in advance of submitting a claim that may be considered fraudulent.

Several sources of coding guidance exist that apply to healthcare facilities as well as professionals that bill for their services. Coding systems vary for healthcare facilities and professionals, as do the reimbursement approaches. Regardless of the coding environment, there remains opportunity for error, either unintentional or intentional. Thus, there is a need for auditing all coding activities.

In addition to CMS's guidelines for coding and reporting, three main regulatory veils exist and should serve to guide healthcare auditing professionals on areas to focus their auditing efforts. Coding professionals should consider these guides and comply with the *Standards for Ethical Coding*. Coding practices will continue to be under the microscope by many from an internal and external perspective given coding's dominant role in reimbursement.

REFERENCES

American Health Lawyers Association (AHLA). n.d. "Corporate Integrity Agreements (CIAs)." Retrieved from *https://www.healthlawyers.org/hlresources/Health%20Law%20Wiki/Corporate%20 Integrity%20Agreements%20(CIAs).aspx.*

Bryant, G. H. 2017. "AHIMA's Revised Standards of Ethical Coding Available." Retrieved from *http:// bok.ahima.org/doc?oid=302300#.WkQC798m7J4.*

CMS. n.d. FAQ on 1995 & 1997 Documentation Guidelines for Evaluation & Management Services. Retrieved from *https://www.cms.gov/Medicare/Medicare-Fee-for-Service-Payment/PhysicianFee-Sched/Downloads/EM-FAQ-1995-1997.pdf.*

CMS. 2007. Civil False Claims Act. Retrieved from *https://downloads.cms.gov/cmsgov/ archived-downloads/SMDL/downloads/SMD032207Att2.pdf*

CMS. 2018. National Correct Coding Initiative Edits. Retrieved from *https://www.cms.gov/Medi-care/Coding/NationalCorrectCodInitEd/index.html?redirect=/nationalcorrectcodinited/.*

Dunn, R.T. 2016. JustCoding's Practical Guide to Coding Management. Middleton, MA: HCPro, Inc., 2016.

Office of Inspector General (OIG). n.d.a. Work Plan. Retrieved from *https://oig.hhs.gov/ reports-and-publications/workplan/.*

Office of Inspector General (OIG). n.d.b. Corporate Integrity Agreements. Retrieved from *https:// oig.hhs.gov/compliance/corporate-integrity-agreements/index.asp.*

Palmetto GBA. 2016. "Differences between 1995 and 1997 E/M Documentation Guide-lines." Retrieved from *https://www.palmettogba.com/palmetto/providers.nsf/DocsCat/ Providers~Railroad%20Medicare~Resources~FAQs~EM%20Help%20Center~8EELQC1460.*

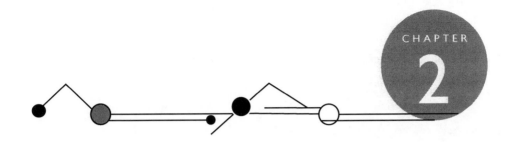

Conducting Coding Audits

CHAPTER OBJECTIVES

- Identify the goals of the coding audit
- Discuss topics to be reviewed
- Address the reasons for conducting coding audits

Why We Should Conduct Coding Audits

A coding audit may be conducted by internal staff or external entities, typically representing the insurers paying for the care. When planning to implement a coding auditing program, the type of reviews, focus areas, and review frequency must all be taken into consideration, as each facet impacts the level of staffing required to conduct the reviews.

The three primary goals for conducting coding reviews are to:

- Identify opportunities for coder and provider education
- Support the organization's revenue integrity initiatives
- Enhance the revenue cycle by ensuring accurate claims are submitted and not subject to coding rejections and denials

If these goals are achieved, the organization should be successful in defending its coding practices with external auditors.

If we look at each of the elements of a coding audit previously described, we can see the benefits that coding reviews provide an organization. Every healthcare organization, including home health agencies, physician practices, ambulatory surgery centers, skilled nursing facilities, and hospitals, should invest in routine, internal coding audits. The alternative is waiting until the payer conducts an audit, denies a claim, and incurs costs for an organization.

When we assess the accuracy of the codes assigned, we will be able to identify the competencies of our coding team to:

- Appropriately seek clarification through the creating and content of physician queries.

- Distinguish clinical indications that identify the presence of an underlying and/or undocumented condition.

- Apply *Coding Clinic,* the *ICD-10-CM/PCS Official Guidelines for Coding and Reporting,* and other industry-recognized guidelines (American Medical Association's [AMA] *CPT Assistant* and *CPT-4® Manual,* National Correct Coding Initiative, etc.) to accurately code conditions and procedures. During this portion of the assessment, the auditor will also determine whether the coder is avoiding the coding of redundant conditions or conditions that are part of the definitive diagnosis or implied by the primary diagnosis, but able to distinguish symptoms or conditions that should be coded because they will support medical necessity.

- Select the principal diagnosis or reason for the encounter and properly sequence secondary conditions.

- Capture all relevant conditions that should be coded to accurately reflect the severity of the patient's condition being treated.

Leveraging the Coding Review

However, coding reviews also provide an opportunity for you to conduct a thorough compliance review that not only addresses other components of the coding process but also the integrity of the patient's record, including but not limited to:

Accuracy of present-on-admission (POA) assignment: The POA code may affect reimbursement. If a condition was present at the time of admission, then the organization may not be faulted for it in the quality measurement system, and reimbursement should remain as anticipated. However, if a condition arises during an encounter, such as a pressure ulcer or never event, reimbursement could be decreased accordingly, and the quality measurement system will reflect the situation arising on the organization's watch.

Nursing's assignment of discharge disposition: The discharge disposition may signal whether the reimbursement for the encounter should be shared with another organization that will be providing additional and continued care for the patient, such as a discharge/transfer to a rehabilitation center. If the auditor finds that one or more nurses are incorrectly assigning the discharge disposition, or that the coding specialist is not catching their errors, then an educational opportunity is available. The coding auditor or health information management director along with the patient financial services director and compliance officer should arrange with the chief nursing officer to provide a nursing in-service program for the nursing staff that addresses the importance of accurate disposition assignment and explain how it impacts receiving accurate reimbursement.

Presence of documentation conflicts (directional, condition, etc.): Identifying this situation (e.g., radiology exam states left lung nodule but the surgeon's note states right lung nodule) speaks to the integrity of the data in the patient's record, but it also could identify the need to focus on support services such as transcription. Additionally, if documentation conflicts are caught concurrently, a never event or patient care error may be avoided.

Use and misuse of copy-forward functionality: The copy-forward functionality can be beneficial for clinicians in capturing a complete description of a patient's condition; however, it can be misused. An example I experienced was when a resident used the copy-forward functionality for 17 years of radiology exams. This obviously added bloat to the record and provided no added value. Using the copy-forward functionality for a complete prior encounter to serve as the only documentation for a current encounter could be considered a fraudulent practice and explains why copy-forward is one of the issues included in the Office of Inspector General *Work Plan.*

Untimely documentation, including the creation of documentation all at one time: This would be an observation that the auditor may make when assessing whether documentation was present at the time of coding. If he or she sees that multiple entries or dictated reports are prepared by or for a clinician all on the same date, then this would be a concern that should be shared with the compliance department and possibly the chief medical officer.

Lost clinic data integrity and revenue integrity opportunities resulting from unanswered queries or queries not issued: As inferred, this situation would occur when a physician query was not issued or has gone unanswered. If the query had been issued or answered, there may have been more specificity in describing a condition or procedure that may have resulted in a higher-weighted hierarchical condition category (HCC) or diagnosis-related group.

The need to modify e-forms and/or templates: An example of this is when the coding auditor notices a trend with one or more clinicians failing to provide a certain element required for coding, such as chronicity. In this case, chronicity may be added to the e-form or template as a way to prompt the physician to select acute, chronic, or other choices. Another example is when the clinician does not complete all fields of an e-form or template. In this situation, the auditor may suggest to information technology that one or more fields must be required fields.

Incorrect charges: One area where auditing can demonstrate immediate fiscal value is when the audit identifies missed charges or mischarges.

- Missed charges occur when a service is documented but no charge appears on the detailed claim. This may have resulted from a lost charge ticket, no-charge code for the service, or the human error of failing to charge for a service.

- Mischarges may be observed when there is a charge on the detailed claim that is clearly in error or when the system autopopulated a charge. An example of an obvious error is a charge for the obstetrical suite for a man. A system-generated charge may occur when a physician does a joint injection and the charge system options provide only the code that is associated with ultrasound guidance. In this case, the physician would routinely be charging for an injection with ultrasound guidance when such guidance was not used.

- Auditors may also capture charge entry error rates when conducting charge-related audits. When the missed charge is due to human error, it would be attributed to the designated charge entry technician. Similarly, if the male patient is assigned the obstetric suite charge, the mischarge would be attributed to the charge entry technician.

Chargemaster-related issues: These issues may surface in denial investigations as well as scrubber edits. They may surface when charges are duplicated on the claim, when charges are missing from the claim, or, as in our injection example above, when charges are incorrectly reported on the claim. They may also be observed during a charge audit when the auditor notes that a soft code is hard coded in the charge description master.

- Soft coding is also known as dynamic coding and should occur when a coder reviews a service. This typically happens with a surgical service; after distinguishing certain conditions present during the surgery, the coder is able to apply the correct code from the several options given. An example would be laparoscopy. In order to know which code to assign when a laparoscopy is performed, the coder reads the procedure report to determine whether it was a diagnostic laparoscopy or a surgical laparoscopy, whether there were specimens collected, how the specimens were collected, whether there were associated procedures, such as an aspiration or drainage procedure, and so on. Each refinement of this procedure may yield a different code.

- Hard codes are static. They are assigned to procedures that are clearly defined, for example, urinalysis by dip stick (CPT code 81000) and an automated urinalysis with microscopy (CPT code 81001). When the order is placed for this test, the specimen is handled according to the order.

Validation of the hours for observations and infusions: Both of these audit topics have a fiscal value and are typically identified as educational opportunities. Correctly counting the hours of observation requires an understanding of those services that may be included in the hour count. This is in contrast to the time documented for other services that must be deducted from the hour count, otherwise known as "carveout" time. Carveouts may include other procedures that are composed of active monitoring as part of the procedure, such as colonoscopies or chemotherapy. Infusion issues surface when the clinician states "infusion" but the infusion services documented lack the start and stop times; therefore, the services must be coded as a push rather than an infusion. When this occurs, there is a loss of revenue. Both situations lend themselves to teaching opportunities, the former with either the coding or billing team and the latter with the nursing staff.

According to Debbie Rubio, BS, MT (ASCP), manager of regulatory affairs and compliance at Medical Management Plus, Inc., "observation time begins at the clock time documented in the patient's medical record, which coincides with the time that observation care is initiated in accordance with a physician's order."

What does this mean exactly? First, there must be a physician's order for observation before observation services can begin. Observation orders cannot be back-dated. For example, when condition code 44 is used to change a patient's status from inpatient to outpatient, observation services do not begin until there is an order for observation (which would be after the change to outpatient status). Observation services would begin at the time that order was written.

If the patient is already actively receiving care, such as in the example above, then observation begins at the time the observation order is written. For patients being transferred to a room after an observation order is written, observation care may not begin until the patient begins to receive evaluation and/or care in the hospital room (Rubio, 2016).

Dating, timing, and signing practices: Particularly important for HCC audits is attention to the Risk Adjustment Validation audit criteria. This includes having a valid clinician signature, credentials, date, and time on each piece of documentation used for coding purposes.

Informed consent validation: This is especially important given CMS' informed consent initiatives (Kelly, 2017). This review focuses on the presence of clinical documentation but is unrelated to coding. It is incorporated in this list as it is an easy "add-on" to do when reviewing surgical encounters.

Presence of patient identifiers on each page: This is another element that is particularly important for physician practices being reimbursed under an HCC model.

Abbreviation usage: Use of "do not use" abbreviations as well as abbreviations that have not been approved for use by your organization can be assessed during an audit. This is another add-on that often falls on the shoulders of coding specialists. Since the coding specialists are reading the record, they often see abbreviations being used that may not be on the approved abbreviation list or may be an abbreviation that is on the "do not use" list. These cases should be flagged. However, the same should occur when the coding compliance auditors are reviewing records and their observation of these unorthodox uses should be tracked and reported.

Presence of more than one patient in a record: This situation is also often an additional responsibility for the coding specialists and should be part of the clinical integrity responsibility of the coding auditor. Observations of mixed files should be reported to the compliance department, privacy officer, and release of information department. The privacy officer should be notified if the record had been released to anyone, thus presenting a breach for one of the patients. The situation is reported to compliance to assess whether patient care may have been negatively affected by the mixed patient information.

Presence of mis-scanned or poorly scanned documents: This last item is similar to the mixed-patient record issue discussed above. If another patient's document was mis-scanned into the record or if a document was mis-scanned to the wrong area of the patient's record, it may have patient care implications. If there is a quality issue with the scanning, such as the documents are skewed, upside down, without patient identifiers, or not clear, there may be patient care implications. Both situations may require additional education for the scanning technicians.

Coding compliance audits cannot cover each of these points in a single audit. The effort to select the sample that encompasses each of these factors and the time to review each for the presence or absence of the attribute would be tremendous. Auditors should pick a few key elements to review, and the items should be of importance to your organization. Ideally, the topics will focus on issues that are frequent or require reassurance. Repeated denials for the sequencing of principal diagnoses may be alarming, but an audit may reveal that the coding specialists are doing their best to comply with the various coding guidelines. However, some coding audits should be routinely scheduled to assess the status quo, that is, whether the coding is being done accurately and completely for a random sample of cases, regardless of the diagnoses or clinicians involved.

Summary

In essence, the objective of conducting coding audits should be to ensure the completeness and accuracy of coding and coding-related processes as well as to identify any issues with the integrity and completeness of the documentation. While many audits are performed solely to improve reimbursement, when audits have a purpose of improving performance, improved reimbursement may occur by default.

REFERENCES

Kelly, T. 2017. "HIM Challenges: Sweeping Change Coming to Informed Consent." For the Record, Vol. 29, No. 11, p.10. Retrieved from *http://www.fortherecordmag.com/archives/1117p10.shtml.*

Rubio, D. 2016. "Counting Observation Hours." Medical Management Plus Inc. Retrieved from *http://www.mmplusinc.com/news-articles/item/counting-observation-hours.*

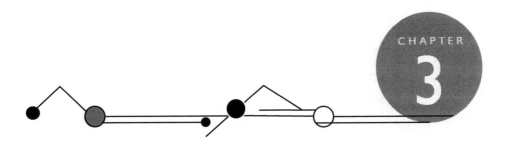

Types of Coding Audits

CHAPTER OBJECTIVES

- Discuss the attributes of a coding audit

- Review the qualifications of a coding compliance auditor candidate

- Distinguish the roles of the internal coding auditor from the external coding auditor

- Discuss the focus areas for key governmental auditors and governmental entities

- Explore the role of the internal coding compliance auditor in relation to external auditors

The Purpose of the Audit

Audits are performed for different purposes by individuals within and outside of an organization. The goal of the audit will vary based on purpose. Audits can be categorized in a variety of ways as shown below, but these attributes are not exclusive: Audits will have several characteristics at a time.

Audits can be categorized in the following ways:

- By the entity that conducts them, for example, by internal staff or external staff

- By purpose, such as compliance purposes, educational purposes, due diligence (such as an entity acquisition or merger), to explain variations in the case-mix index, to update problem lists for active and inactive conditions, to investigate reported trends from external agencies (such as the Comprehensive Error Rate Testing or The Program for Evaluating Payment Patterns Electronic Report [PEPPER]), and more

- By topic, for example, by hierarchal condition category, evaluation and management codes (E/M), diagnosis-related groups (DRG), present-on-admission codes, abbreviation usage, etc.

- For identifying trends, such as the following: physician response rate to queries; documentation timeliness; lack of dates, times, or signatures; legibility; coding errors by coder; use of unspecified codes; disposition errors by patient care floor or nurse; consistency between clinical documentation improvement and coding teams; etc.

- For the benefit of the healthcare organization or benefit of the payers

In this chapter, we will discuss audits in terms of the entity that conducts them. Internal audits are conducted by employees of the organization, while external audits are conducted by individuals who may be engaged by the healthcare organization or engaged or employed by another entity to assess the healthcare organization.

Internal Audits

In the earlier chapters, we have discussed the reason for coding audits. One of our objectives is to ensure our coding is supported by the documentation in the patient's record, but we may also include other elements to address while we are looking at the audit.

Internal reviewers

Internal audits should be conducted by individuals with honed coding skills and whose coding opinions are respected by others on the coding team. Often, the coding compliance auditors are employees of the coding department. While it is common for a supervisor or lead coder to conduct the reviews, some organizations hire a person whose sole job is to conduct coding audits. Larger organizations may have separate departments that solely perform coding audits. The separate departments may evaluate the coding performed by the health information management (HIM) coding team, the physician practice coding, coding by other patient support areas, such as interventional radiology or physical therapy, and the charge description master coding.

Being a coding auditor should not be an "other duties as required" assignment. However, there are coding audit approaches that suggest using peers as coding auditors, especially when the peers perform the same type of coding. In this context, the "auditing" is more of a "collaborative validation." This approach is commonly used by external auditors conducting coding and accounting audits and also is known as interrater reliability. This means that each "rater" or auditor assesses the case and then compares their assessments. If their determinations differ, the case is discussed until the two auditors agree on what the preferred decision should be. Interrating continues until the auditors have a predetermination agreement rate. The practice may be that they agree on their determinations for five consecutive cases or 10% of the cases. Doing this approach ensures that the individuals' determinations made for the remaining cases will be reliably consistent. When used in a "collaborative validation" environment and there is consistent agreement between the two colleagues, then a third individual may need to spot check the coding to ensure there is a collegial consensus and make sure routine acceptance of each other's coding is not occurring.

Depending on the environment and type of coding performed, individuals with different expertise and/or credentials or certifications will conduct the reviews. For example, an individual reviewing professional coding may have a Certified Coding Specialist—Physician-based (CCS-P), Certified Professional Coder (CPC), or Certified Risk Adjustment Coder (CRC) certification, while an individual reviewing inpatient hospital coding may have a Certified Coding Specialist (CCS) certification. Regardless of the credentials or certifications, the key characteristics of the individual performing the reviews are expertise and communication skills. An auditor that thrives on "gotcha" results will not be respected, nor will the auditor be effective in achieving the outcomes we expect from audits—improved performance. His or her actions will only create an environment where team members are on edge or fearful of the auditor's intent. Coders could become dissatisfied with their work environment and leave for other opportunities. Coding professionals are too difficult to recruit to encourage them to leave because of an individual with a "gotcha" attitude.

The preferred approach and attitude is as an "educator/collaborator." A coder will be more receptive when approached by an auditor who says:

> *I see you chose this code. I can't find the documentation that supported it. Could you show me where you found it? I did find this piece of Dr. X's progress note, and that led me to recommending this code instead. What do you think?*

I employ a large team of coding professionals and they often tell me that coding is not always black and white. An auditor that uses a collaborative approach will attempt to gain consensus from those being audited. In doing so, the auditor must be able to identify those coding rules or guidelines that apply to the situation, share them with those being audited, and clearly explain (educator characteristic) why the application of the specific rule or guideline favors the auditor's choice in code(s).

Coding compliance auditor or liaison?

The coding compliance auditor may serve as the coding team's liaison with others in the organization, such as clinical documentation improvement, quality or performance management, core measures, case management, and patient financial services. The liaison role does not differ significantly from the role the auditor plays with the coding team.

In the liaison role, he or she is responding to coding-related questions such as "Why was this coded this way?" The rationale often lies in a coding guideline that will be shared with the inquirer. There may be the need to debate whether other code options should be used based on clinical evidence and payer requirements. The ability to diplomatically and authoritatively support the coding rationale is important for the coding compliance auditor.

Coding compliance auditor characteristics and skills

The auditor candidate must be well versed in coding rules and practice and have attention to detail, but they may also need some noncoding skills, such as:

- Reporting design, knowing what data needs to be pulled and how it should be displayed
- Report writing, the ability to pull in the data and select a random sample of cases
- Database and spreadsheet (e.g., Access, Excel, etc.) skills, the ability to develop reports using pivot tables and display data in graph formats
- Writing skills, the ability to create the summary of the findings
- Interpersonal skills, understanding that the role should nurture collaborative and cooperative relations with other revenue cycle departments and coworkers within the department
- Teaching skills, the ability to convey rationale and new concepts to the coding team at different learning levels or in terms that can be assimilated by the team members

- Presentation skills, the ability to share results and respond to ad hoc questions from the coding team, department management, compliance committee, and senior leadership

When selecting an individual to perform the coding auditing function for your organization, the incumbent's noncoding skills should be considered. Some of these skills may be learned while on the job, such as spreadsheet use and report writing. Others, however, should be apparent in the candidate's demeanor, writing, and interview responses before selecting an individual. An example of a position description for a coding compliance auditor appears in the downloadable appendix of this book.

Why do internal audits?

As discussed in Chapter 2, there are three goals for conducting coding reviews:

1. Identify opportunities for coder and provider education

2. Support the organization's revenue integrity initiatives

3. Enhance the revenue cycle by ensuring accurate claims are submitted and not subject to coding rejections and denials

Discussion of coding audit findings on a frequent basis throughout the year reinforces adult learning. Coding correctly is based on an understanding of the rules, ability to apply the rules to the scenario, and practice. Just like habits may take a few months of repetition to develop, so does correct coding. Doing frequent audits will continue to reinforce correct coding expectations with the coding and professional teams more effectively than only conducting an annual review.

Only conducting annual reviews fails to sufficiently reinforce habits. If there is no reinforcement of the audit findings with staff involved, then some (or all) errors may continue, which does not support the goal to ensure revenue integrity nor contribute to the revenue cycle's success in creating clean and accurate claims that reduce denials. In summary, an organization that wishes to achieve revenue cycle effectiveness and efficiency must conduct coding reviews throughout the year.

External Audits

External audits may be performed by an individual or firm that is hired by the healthcare organization or by a third party that is not associated with the healthcare organization. When the healthcare organization engages an individual or firm to conduct the audit, the audit should be considered "for the benefit" of the healthcare organization. The focus of the audit conducted by a firm that is hired by the healthcare organization may be similar to those we discussed earlier. Often, these contracted audit engagements are more extensive and cover multiple aspects or conditions that may have surfaced during the internal reviews or common industry challenges that the consultant is seeing in other organizations.

The consultant will provide a written report of findings and coding accuracy rates as well as provide citations (official sources) for some of the changes recommended. Additionally, the consultant will usually provide an educational session for the coders, providers, clinical documentation improvement staff, and/or compliance teams based on the findings. The key findings are areas that may need to be reinforced through follow-up audits conducted by the internal auditing team to ensure the educational message conveyed by the consultant was understood and is being applied.

When the external auditor is employed by an entity other than the healthcare organization, the benefit of the audit is primarily for that other entity. Other entities are typically governmental or commercial payers, but entities may also be a buyer that is contemplating merging with or acquiring the healthcare organization or a rating agency that is assessing the healthcare organization's financial strength for loan or bond purposes. These audits will focus on the external entity's interests. For governmental or commercial payers, it will be primarily on claims they paid and patterns they saw while adjudicating the claims. For entities considering a merger or acquisition, they will be focusing on the financial strength and related financial risks of the organization. Obviously, the accuracy of coding will be a critical concern of theirs as well as the overall efficiency and effectiveness of each of the departments within the revenue cycle.

Several governmental external auditors and entities that monitor coding are described below (Dunn, 2016).

Comprehensive Error Rate Testing

Managed by CMS, the Comprehensive Error Rate Testing (CERT) program was established to monitor the accuracy of claim payments in the Medicare Fee-For-Service program.

The intent of the CERT program is to protect the Medicare Trust Fund by identifying errors and assessing error rates at both the national and regional levels. In essence, the CERT measures improper payments. Findings from the CERT program are used to identify trends that are driving the errors, such as errors by a specific provider type or service, and to assist with allocation of future program integrity resources. The CERT program is recognized as one that alerts providers of trends noticed from providers' billings. When a provider receives a trend report from the CERT, it should seriously evaluate its coding practices. The CERT error rate is also used by CMS to evaluate and measure the performance of Medicare contractors.

Annually, the Department of Health and Human Services (HHS) reviews their programs to improve agency efforts to reduce and recover improper payments. When improper payments are identified, HHS or CMS may use contractors, such as the Recovery Audit Contractors (RAC), to investigate and recover those improper payments. Improper payments are not limited to overpayments, since underpayments may be identified by the program reviews as well. When an underpayment is identified, contractors may be used to investigate and, when appropriate, take action to have a refund issued.

Improper payments include:

- Payments to an ineligible recipient
- Payments for an ineligible service
- Duplicate payments (more than one payment for the same service)
- Payments for services that were not received
- Payments for an incorrect amount

Many ask how the government, after all these years of processing claims, could make some of these improper payments, e.g., payments for an ineligible service or recipient.

When improper payment claims are reviewed, the common categories identified are:

- No or insufficient documentation
- Medical necessity
- Incorrect coding
- Other

Three of the above-listed categories fall into the coding professional's realm.

No or insufficient documentation: Sometimes codes are submitted from an encounter form or superbill rather than being based on the documentation in the progress or encounter note (see Figure 3.1). These check-off documents are often segregated from the actual medical record documentation. Coding professionals should code from the source medical record and use the superbill or encounter form as a guide. If the documentation does not support the conditions or services checked off, then the provider should be queried.

FIGURE 3.1 ENCOUNTER FORM EXAMPLE

	John J. Smith, MD Geneticist 948 Apple Lane, Apple Valley (314) 555-4444				
DIAGNOSIS & FINDINGS					
P09	Neonatal Screening	Q18.9	Dysmorphic Features	R56.9	Seizure Disorder
Q77.4	Achondroplasia	R62.51	Failure to Thrive	Q97.0	Karyotype 47,XXX
E87.2	Acidosis	Z84.81	Family History of Genetic Disorder	Q97.2	Mosaicism-various # X Chromosomes
P84	Acidosis of Newborn			Q97.3	Female w 46,XY Karyotype
Q56.4	Ambiguous Genitalia	R01.0	Heart Murmur, Benign & Innocent	Q98.5	Karyotype 47,XYY
F84.0	Autism	R01.1	Heart Murmur, Unspecified	Q99.8	Other Chromosomal Anomaly, Specified
Q99.9	Chromosome Abnormality	R00.8	Heart Beat, Other abnormality	R62.52	Short Stature (Pediatric)
Q36.9	Cleft Lip, Unilateral	Q54.9	Hypospadias	Q91.7	Trisomy 13
Q93.89	Other Deletions-Autosomes	P05.10	Newborn Small for Gestational Age	Z31.430	Testing Female for Disease Carrier Status Encounter
R62.0	Delayed Milestones	Q87.1	Noonan Syndrome	Z31.438	Other Genetic Testing Female for Procreative Mgmt. Encounter

Other Services: _____

_____

Provider's Signature: _____

Date: _____

Source: Rose T. Dunn. Reprinted with permission.

Medical necessity: When receptionists register a patient for a clinical test, the condition for which the test is being conducted should be assessed for its support of medical necessity. The assessment may be accomplished by using medical necessity software that is often integrated in the electronic health record used by the organization. When the conditions on the order do not support the test, either the ordering provider's office is called for additional clarification or the patient is notified that the service may not be paid for by the payers. When this occurs, the patient is notified in writing and asked to sign an acknowledgment that they may be having a test for which they will be financially responsible for the cost.

However, there are times when the coder is completing the coding function and may receive an alert from the encoder or the billing scrubber that the condition coded for an outpatient service does not meet medical necessity. The coder's obligation is to re-review the documentation to determine whether other conditions were documented either in the physician notes or order as related to the test or service.

Incorrect coding: This may mean that incorrect (possibly related to an NCCI edit) or outdated code(s) were applied to the claim by a coder, coder-biller, or provider, or that the service codes selected by the service department from the charge-description master are incorrect or were not accurately selected.

When the latter two conditions start increasing in frequency, therefore resulting in delayed claims awaiting attention by the coding team, the internal auditor should take note and focus his or her attention on who initially coded the encounter, if there is an outdated code in the charge-description master, or if someone's encoder has not been updated, and who the physician is. The latter is an important piece of the puzzle, because occasionally physicians supply codes for tests ordered and for procedures scheduled. Sometimes, these codes are incorrect. If the codes are entered into the system, bypass the coder, and then reject when they are processed through the scrubber, physician education may be required.

Program for Evaluating Payment Patterns Electronic Report

Texas Medical Foundation is contracted with CMS, to develop, produce, and disseminate the Program for Evaluating Payment Patterns Electronic Report (PEPPER) (Texas Medical Foundation, n.d.). PEPPER provides provider-specific Medicare data statistics for discharges/services vulnerable to improper payments. The statistics are based on the claim data from your facility. PEPPER can support a hospital or facility's compliance efforts by identifying where it is an outlier for these risk areas. These data can help identify both potential overpayments as well as potential underpayments. While PEPPER is not necessarily an auditor, the data it collects may be used by external auditing agencies.

PEPPER summarizes your hospital's Medicare claims data statistics and compares them with aggregate Medicare data from other hospitals in the nation, in your Medicare Administrative Contractor (MAC) jurisdiction, and in the state. These comparisons are the first step in identifying where your hospital's statistics might differ from the majority of other providers and could be an indication of higher risk for improper Medicare payments, possibly due to coding. These reports are available for providers other than short-term acute care facilities, including critical access hospitals, home health agencies, hospices, inpatient psychiatric facilities, inpatient rehabilitation facilities, long-term acute care hospitals, partial hospitalization programs, and skilled nursing facilities.

The coding compliance auditor can utilize the data from the PEPPER to:

- Identify potential DRG overcoding and undercoding
- Identify DRGs that are problematic on which the hospital or facility may want to focus auditing and monitoring
- Access tables and graphs displaying billing activity over time in comparison with other hospitals or facilities, which can be used for educational training activities
- Prioritize areas for coding compliance auditing and monitoring
- Aid efforts to improve medical record documentation

MACs

The MACs are the consolidation of the former fiscal intermediaries (Part A) and carriers (Part B). By consolidating all provider components in several regional claim processing entities, MACs have access to all provider claims, are able to see the entire episode of care and services provided by all its players, can follow hospital disposition errors including "unknowns," and are able to surface hospital/physician inconsistency in diagnosis codes, e.g., excisional debridement billed by the physician versus a nonexcisional debridement billed by the hospital.

These findings can trigger a RAC investigation, but often the MAC utilizes its own staff or the Quality Improvement Organization (QIO). The RAC reviews both inpatient and outpatient claims with a focus on recovering improper payments made by the MACs or other governmental entities. The QIO focuses on inpatient hospital claims with a goal to prevent improper payments of DRG assignments by hospitals.

Similarly, the MAC's focus is to prevent future improper payments (before payment), thus the reason for prepay holds. With the consolidated claim database, the MACs are able to identify suspected billing problems, inconsistencies, and aberrancies and place the respective providers on a prepay hold or ask another governmental agency to investigate. Some of the trends identified by the MAC trigger the CERT notice that we discussed earlier.

The Office of Inspector General

The Office of Inspector General (OIG) has a broad reach in terms of enforcement and has the right to "look back" over 10 years. The OIG focuses on identifying fraud and monitors payers, providers, governmental agencies, and governmental contractors. The OIG maintains the Excluded Individuals and Entities List, which identifies individuals and entities who have submitted false, fraudulent, or otherwise improper claims for Medicare or Medicaid payment.

Additionally, the OIG monitors interprovider activities, such as ordering patterns between physicians, home health, and pharmaceutical companies, and monitors the effectiveness of organizations' compliance programs. While the OIG investigates complaints, it may engage another agency or contractor to take action.

Risk Adjustment Data Validation Contractors

Risk Adjustment Data Validation Contractors (RADV) focus on the accuracy of claims submitted for patients who are covered by the Medicare Advantage program. Specifically, they review claims the Medicare Advantage Health Plan submits to CMS. Since the health plan is reimbursed by CMS on a hierarchal condition category basis (which is driven by the acute and chronic conditions being treated or monitored by the physician), the accuracy of the reported conditions is paramount. These reviewers assess not only whether the condition is supported in the documentation but also whether the documentation meets the requirements to be considered as supportive of the condition. They review for authentication of the documentation (signature and credentials) and other elements. The RADV checklist could be used as an auditing tool (see Figures 3.2A and 3.2B). More detailed RADV guidance is available in the CMS publication "Contract-Level Risk Adjustment Data Validation Medical Record Reviewer Guidance As of 9/27/17."

FIGURE 3.2A RADV CHECKLIST

1

Centers for Medicare & Medicaid Services
Risk Adjustment Data Validation (RADV) Medical Record Checklist and Guidance

This checklist list was provided to plans involved in the calendar year (CY) 2009 and CY 2010 national RADV audits. This list may help to determine a record's suitability for Risk Adjustment Data Validation (RADV). Any items checked "no" may indicate that the record will not support a CMS-HCC.

Yes   No

☐   ☐   **Is the record for the correct enrollee?**

☐   ☐   **Is the record from the correct calendar year for the payment year being audited (i.e., for audits of 2011 payments, validating records should be from calendar year 2010)**

☐   ☐   **Is the date of service present for the face to face visit?**

☐   ☐   **Is the record legible?**

☐   ☐   **Is the record from a valid provider type?** (Hospital inpatient, hospital outpatient/ physician)

☐   ☐   **Are there valid credentials and/or is there a valid physician specialty documented on the record?**

☐   ☐   **Does the record contain a signature from an acceptable type of physician specialist?**

☐   ☐   **If the outpatient/physician record does not contain a valid credential and/or signature, is there a completed CMS-Generated Attestation for this date of service?**

☐   ☐   **Is there a diagnosis on the record?**

☐   ☐   **Does the diagnosis support an HCC?**

☐   ☐   **Does the diagnosis support the requested HCC?**

Information contained in this document is intended to provide general guidelines for representatives of Medicare Advantage (MA) contracts selected for Risk Adjustment Data Validation (RADV). The guidance provided here does not guarantee that the documentation that you submit for review will validate the HCC under review. The Centers for Medicare & Medicaid Services (CMS) may determine the validity of medical record documentation based on criteria other than those described herein. Submission of medical record documentation for RADV must comply with all CMS instructions.

FIGURE 3.2B RADV CHECKLIST

2

Centers for Medicare & Medicaid Services
Risk Adjustment Data Validation (RADV) Medical Record Checklist and Guidance

When submitting a record for RADV, consider the following:

- If the condition warrants an inpatient hospitalization, the HCC may be supported by an inpatient record. Examples of such conditions may include septicemia, cerebral hemorrhage, cardio respiratory failure, and shock. For these conditions, an inpatient record, a stand-alone inpatient consultation record, or a stand-alone discharge summary may be appropriate for submission.

- When possible, obtain a record from the specialist treating the condition, e.g. an oncologist for a cancer diagnosis. These records may be more likely to sufficiently document the condition.

- Pay special attention to cancer diagnoses. A notation indicating "history of cancer," without an indication of current cancer treatment, may not be sufficient documentation for validation. For example, if in an attempt to validate HCC 10 (Breast, Prostate, Colorectal and Other Cancers and Tumors) a Medicare Advantage contract submits a record that indicates a patient has a history of cancer that was last treated outside the data collection year, the HCC may be not be validated.

- When reviewing medical records, pay special attention to the problem list on electronic medical records. Often, in certain systems, a diagnosis never drops off the list, even if the patient is no longer suffering from the condition. Conversely, the problem list may not document the HCC your MA contract submitted for payment.

- Any problem list in submitted documentation should be included and not just referenced.

- Records submitted to validate HCCs that encompass additional manifestations or complications related to the disease (e.g. HCC 15, Diabetes with Renal Manifestations or Diabetes with Peripheral Circulatory Manifestations) should include language from an acceptable physician specialist which establishes a causal link between the disease and the complication. An acceptable record that clearly defines the complication or manifestation and expressly relates it to the disease may validate the HCC. A record that does not define and link this relationship may not validate the HCC.

- If a physician or outpatient record is missing a provider's signature and/or credentials, consider using the CMS-Generated Attestation that was provided with your data. CMS will only consider CMS-Generated Attestations for RADV.

- Minimum requirements for inpatient records state that these must contain an admission and discharge date. In addition
  - inpatient records must include the signed discharge summary,
  - stand-alone consultations must contain the consultation date, and
  - stand-alone discharge summaries submitted as physician provider type must contain the discharge date

Information contained in this document is intended to provide general guidelines for representatives of Medicare Advantage (MA) contracts selected for Risk Adjustment Data Validation (RADV). The guidance provided here does not guarantee that the documentation that you submit for review will validate the HCC under review. The Centers for Medicare & Medicaid Services (CMS) may determine the validity of medical record documentation based on criteria other than those described herein. Submission of medical record documentation for RADV must comply with all CMS instructions.

RACs

The RACs are also regionally assigned and have access to all provider claims, and they focus on quality of care, medical necessity, and preserving the Medicare Trust Fund. The RACs post the topics that their investigations will address.

As such, the RACs focus on detecting and recovering improper payments. Some of the RAC coding focus areas include:

- DRG validation
- Units of services or medication on the claim
- E/M codes: frequency on same day, location, and new versus established patients
- Outpatient and inpatient services that may be being "abused" (medical necessity)
- Discharge disposition reporting
- Two qualifying principal diagnoses
- Violations of Medicare's global surgery payment rules even in cases involving E/M services
- E/M services that are not reasonable and necessary

The RACs have been successful in returning improper payments back to the Medicare Trust Fund. The RACs have been compensated under an incentive-driven payment system.

Zone Program Integrity Contractors

The Zone Program Integrity Contractors (ZPIC) are another layer of investigatory and enforcement contractors. They receive referrals from the RACs and other agencies. ZPICs focus on fraud identification and investigations and target durable medical equipment companies, physical therapists, and physicians who order these services. As part of the investigation, the contractor can request an unlimited number of records and can place a provider on 100% prebill hold. The ZPICs investigate all fraud leads and monitor the internet and news to surface provider irregularities. If the ZPIC investigation substantiates fraud, the case is referred to the OIG. The OIG can apply both civil and criminal prosecution and sanctions.

The Medicaid Integrity Contractor

The Medicaid Integrity Contractor (MIC) serves in a similar capacity as the RACs but only for Medicaid claims. They partner with designated Medicaid RACs as well. The MIC investigations may be more challenging than the RACs in that each state has its own Medicaid program and program rules. They use the payment error rate measurement program to identify providers to review and possibly audit. The MICs focus on education, auditing, and reviews, and unlike RACs, MICs are not paid on a contingency basis.

Healthcare Fraud Prevention and Enforcement Action Team

The Healthcare Fraud Prevention and Enforcement Action Team is a partnership of OIG and the U.S. Department of Justice. They have several cities that are focus cities. Their target is cheaters that are identified through extensive data mining or flagged by other audit entities.

Third-party payers

Third-party payers will conduct random and focused audits of claims that have charges that are unusually high or inconsistent with the conditions reported by the providers. For example, this would happen if all inpatient encounters are level five, if all office encounters with a procedure have an E/M code with a modifier -25, or for claims with conditions that are not covered by the health plan. The MAC may place a provider on prepay review. This means that prior to adjudicating the claim and making payment to the provider, the provider may be required to submit copies of their patient records with the claims for review by the payers prior to payment. The insurers often use sophisticated analytics comparing providers within the same specialty to one another and hospitals of comparable size to other hospitals, to identify trends or peculiarities, similar to how PEPPER identifies variations. Each of the commercial insurers also employs staff members that monitor claims data for aberrations and trends. When indicated, the commercial insurer will conduct its own reviews. We have devoted Chapter 5 to the audit practices of payers in this book.

It should be apparent from the above discussion that there are many organizations involved in assessing the accuracy of codes and claims submitted, in addition to the groups we have discussed in earlier chapters. To keep abreast of audit goals requires regular reviews of the external auditor websites and professional association articles. Some specialty associations publish guidance for their professional members. An example of such guidance is from the American College of Emergency Physicians. This resource, which appears in the appendix of this book, not only identifies what payers are monitoring, but also what information is necessary to prepare an appeal for any denials.

Facilitating External Audits

The coding compliance auditor may be responsible for coordinating external audits. If the external auditor is a payer, the coding compliance auditor should validate that the payer has the right to access the records. This can be accomplished by confirming that the payer is listed on the record or by checking with patient financial services to see if the insurer is a payer on the account. Only accounts for which a payer is responsible should be provided to the external auditor without a patient's explicit authorization.

Next, the coding compliance auditor will collect the records requested by the auditor, ensuring that only those encounters to which the auditor is authorized are collected. Collecting may include pulling the records if paper, queuing the records if electronic, or copying the records if the records are being sent to the external auditor. When the external auditor is not coming on-site, organizations with an electronic health record (EHR) should consider queuing the records to an auditor queue and providing the reviewer with remote access to the queue—only to avoid the cost of duplicating or loading the record to other media. Providing external auditors with access to your EHR while they work on-site is preferred. An auditor's logins and document views are typically tracked in the EHR's access logs, and the queue can be restricted to only the encounters they are authorized to see.

The coding compliance auditor should oversee any coding-related audits that occur on-site. His or her role should include orienting the external auditors to the access route, format of the record, explaining any unique coding practices for the organization, reviewing cases that the external auditors believe are incorrect (including involving the coder who coded the case to obtain the coder's opinion), and, for some external auditors, making copies of requested pages of the record. Finally, the coding compliance auditor may be responsible for coordinating the external auditor's exit meeting and ensuring appropriate individuals are available to meet.

If a final report is issued by the external auditors, as is usually the case for those auditors engaged by the healthcare organization, the coding compliance auditor may be responsible for distributing the report to certain individuals and maintaining the report for the coding compliance files. The final report is a useful tool to use for identifying and planning educational opportunities for the coding team or professional staff and highlighting areas that should be considered for ongoing reviews.

Summary

In this chapter, we have expanded the list of potential external auditors that may be reviewing our coding. In an attempt to mitigate findings, the importance of ongoing coding reviews is emphasized. The role of the coding compliance auditor may be broader than initially thought. The role of the internal coding compliance auditor includes conducting internal audits, providing education, conducting follow-up, managing and monitoring external audits, and serving as a liaison between the coding team and other departments.

REFERENCES

Dunn, R.T. 2016. JustCoding's Practical Guide to Coding Management. Middleton, MA: HCPro, Inc.

Texas Medical Foundation, n.d. "About PEPPER." Retrieved from *https://www.pepperresources.org/ PEPPER.*

CHAPTER 4

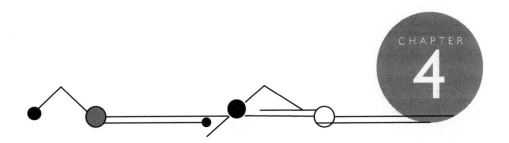

Developing a Coding Compliance Program

CHAPTER OBJECTIVES

- Distinguish between the coding compliance policy and the coding compliance plan
- Define the framework for the coding compliance plan
- Create a coding compliance calendar
- Understand who should receive and how to protect the audit findings

We have discussed who should do coding audits, why coding audits are important, many of the topics that could be audited, and the types of coding audits. Now that we understand these concepts, it is important to develop a written plan for the internal coding compliance program. Doing so is valuable for several reasons:

- Justifying resources allocated to auditing duties
- Demonstrating the coding department efforts to support revenue integrity
- Ensuring consistent and compliant coding performance
- Assisting you in managing the audit effort

When developing a coding compliance program, begin by reviewing any existing coding policies and procedures to determine whether they are consistent with the organization's compliance plan as well as the latest *ICD-10-CM/PCS Official Guidelines for Coding and Reporting* (Dunn, 2016). If your department lacks coding compliance policies and procedures, excellent information on policies and procedures are available at *JustCoding.com, AHIMA.org*, and *HCAHealthcare.com*.

Studying publications from the various regulatory, authoritative, and professional organizations can help managers anticipate what external auditors are observing and targeting. This includes auditors whose services were retained by the facility and auditors from federal agencies and third-party payers. Recognizing vulnerabilities helps identify areas that require evaluation and mitigation.

In this chapter, we will first describe some of the components of a coding policy and plan and then approaches to monitoring coding quality.

Coding Compliance Policy

The policy should be brief but clearly state the reason and scope of the plan. It should be a statement that does not change often. For an example of this, see Figure 4.1. The policy example below can be used for any type of facility by changing a few words and inserting a different title, as shown by the brackets in the statement. The plan itself will be more dynamic than the policy. The plan must be adjusted for new regulations, coding classifications, resources, systems, and so forth.

FIGURE 4.1 POLICY STATEMENT FOR A CODING COMPLIANCE PLAN

Policy: XYZ Physician Practice [ABC Medical Center] intends to abide by federal and payer coding rules. To do so, it will maintain a coding compliance program to periodically review the coding that is applied to claims and the documentation associated with the coding.

The compliance program shall be directed by the compliance officer and implemented by the office manager [HIM director]. External contracted coding consultants will be utilized by the office manager to assist in implementing this program.

Scope: The program will apply to all XYZ Physician Practice [ABC Medical Center] personnel responsible for performing clinical documentation and personnel billing, supervising, recommending, or assigning codes to claims that are submitted to a payer for reimbursement purposes.

Source: Rose T. Dunn. Reprinted with permission.

Coding Compliance Plan

The coding compliance plan may be a subsection of the policy but often is a separate document since it will change periodically. The plan component should be much more detailed and include the specifics of what, when, and how often. Each organization should tailor its coding compliance plan to its organization. When developing a new coding compliance plan, managers should begin by asking these questions:

- Why am I establishing a plan?
- What will I review?
- How will I select a sample?
- How will I assess accuracy?
- What action will I take when the results are known?
- How will I monitor progress?

The coding manager should collaborate with the compliance officer in developing the plan.

Example of a coding compliance plan

The remaining content of this chapter and the example clauses discussed in the next few pages will provide answers to the questions listed above.

Purpose

The purpose of the ABC Medical Center compliance plan is to improve the accuracy and integrity of patient data, ensure minimal variation in coding practices, serve as a conduit to improve provider documentation in the electronic patient record, and support ABC Medical Center's ability to receive its entitled reimbursement for the services it and its providers provide.

Expectation

Staff (employees and, when applicable, contracted staff) will strive to maintain the highest level of professional and ethical standards in the performance of their coding duties. Staff will be trained and oriented in all applicable federal and state laws and regulations that apply to coding and documentation as they relate to their positions. Adherence to these guidelines is imperative. Where any questions or uncertainty regarding these requirements exists, it is the responsibility of the employee to seek guidance from the coding manager, a certified coding specialist, health information management director, or another qualified coding professional. Staff will be familiar with prohibited and unethical conduct that relates to coding and billing as outlined in the facility compliance plan. Staff will comply with AHIMA's *Standards of Ethical Coding*.

Education

All coders, billers, and providers will receive orientation and training in the fundamentals of compliant coding and billing. Continuing education will be provided in the form of handouts, memos, journals, in-services, and formal online and in-person education as available and approved. In order to keep up with changes in regulatory requirements, coding changes, and proper coding procedures, it is the staff member's responsibility to further their knowledge by reading all handouts, memos, and journals provided and actively participate in available in-service and formal education workshops.

All coders, billers, and providers will receive training in coding, documentation, and billing compliance issues on an annual basis or more frequently as need dictates. The training will be coordinated by the coding compliance subcommittee of the compliance committee in conjunction with or in addition to training provided by the compliance office.

Coding resources

Coding staff shall have access to the following resources to facilitate their coding duties:

- Encoder with *Coding Clinic*, AMA's *CPT Assistant*, and other references
- Computer with dual monitors
- Coding books including ICD-10-CM/PCS, CPT-4®, HCPCS, and ProFee coding manuals
- Other references, such as an anatomy and physiology book, interventional radiology reference, *2018 Pocket Guide for Coding Professionals*, *DRG Desk Reference*, etc.
- A compendium of Payer Advisory Notices outlining payer-specific coding expectations and medical necessity rules scanned and/or saved to the coder shared drive

Coding conventions and guidelines

The guidelines and conventions to be followed for codes to be reported on claims will be:

- *Coding Clinic* published by the AHA
- *CPT Assistant* published by the American Medical Association
- The *ICD-10-CM/PCS Official Guidelines for Coding and Reporting* published by CMS and the National Center for Health Statistics

Medicare guidelines

CMS mandates the utilization of Level I (CPT) and Level II (National Medicare) HCPCS codes for Medicare patients. Level III HCPCS codes are created and maintained by the Medicare Administrative Contractors (MAC). It should be noted that Level III HCPCS codes may override Level I or Level II codes; therefore, it is critical to follow MAC coding policies and procedures.

The National Correct Coding Initiative (NCCI) will be strictly adhered to, to identify what is included in a global package and codes that are components of another code to prevent unbundling of services. Claim scrubbers incorporate the NCCI rules when they review the codes reported on the claims to prevent improper payments when incorrect code combinations are reported. The NCCI contains one table of edits for physicians/practitioners and one table of edits for outpatient hospital services.

The official guidelines for specific Medicare coding and billing policies are the *Medicare Part A Manual* and *Medicare Part B Manual, CMS Program Memorandums*, educational events, and MAC newsletters and bulletins. These may be found on the respective MAC websites. A list of current MACs appear in the appendix of this book. The MAC websites will also list their local coverage determinations. However, an alternative resource is the CMS website at *www.cms.gov/medicare-coverage-database*.

UHDDS definitions

Inpatient diagnoses and procedures shall be coded in accordance with Uniform Hospital Discharge Data Set (UHDDS) definitions for principal and additional diagnoses and procedures (CMS, 2012).

Reportable diagnoses and procedures

To achieve consistency in the coding of diagnoses and procedures, coders must follow the *Official Guidelines for Coding and Reporting*, as well as:

- Thoroughly review the entire patient record as part of the coding process in order to assign and report the most appropriate codes.

- Assign and report codes without physician consultation/query for diagnoses and procedures that are not listed in the physician's final diagnostic statement ONLY if those diagnoses and procedures are specifically documented in the body of the patient record by a physician directly participating in the care of the patient and this documentation is clear and consistent. Note: Some organizations specify that in these cases, the diagnoses or procedures must appear more than once in the body of the patient record.

- Areas of the patient record that contain acceptable physician documentation to support code assignment include the discharge summary, history and physical, emergency room record, physician progress notes, physician orders, physician consultations, pathology reports, operative reports, and physician notations of intraoperative occurrences.

- When diagnoses or procedures are stated in other patient record documentation (nurses' notes, radiology reports, laboratory reports, EKGs, nutritional evaluations, or other ancillary reports), the attending physician must be queried for confirmation of the condition (with the exception of the nonphysician provider documentation as outlined below).

- Coders may utilize patient record documentation to provide specificity in coding without querying the physician, such as utilizing the radiology report to confirm the fracture site or referring to the EKG to identify the location of a myocardial infarction.

- Coders may utilize nonphysician provider documentation (nurses' notes or other ancillary provider notes) to specify circumstances and place of occurrence for accidents and injuries when that documentation is omitted by the physician. The coder may code the body mass index (BMI) from the dietitian note, nursing note, or from anywhere in the EMR if documented but ONLY if the physician has documented a diagnosis that goes with the BMI code, such as obesity or malnutrition. If the physician documents a pressure ulcer or decubitus ulcer, the coder may report the stage from the wound care nurses' notes.

- Coders coding in an HCC environment (i.e., for claims submitted to Medicare Advantage, an Accountable Care Organization collaborating with a commercial payer utilizing HCCs as the reimbursement approach, or a Medicaid program using HCCs or for claims submitted to an Affordable Care Act plan), the RADV valid documentation rules apply. Documentation that could be used but is invalid for authentication or patient identity reasons should be referred to the coding manager to address with the appropriate person.

Query process

Utilizing the guidance from the AHIMA's "Guidelines for Achieving a Compliant Query Practice," a coder should query the physician once a diagnosis or procedure has been determined to meet the guidelines for reporting but has not been clearly or completely stated within the patient record by a physician participating in the care of the patient. A query should also be made when questionable, ambiguous, or conflicting documentation is present to determine whether a documented condition was a postoperative complication and for the specific condition for which the patient is receiving medication, therapeutic or diagnostic tests, or treatment (AHIMA, 2016). Additionally, querying should be used to avoid the use of "unspecified" codes.

Each organization should determine whether the query and its response will be maintained in the patient's record or stored elsewhere. If stored elsewhere, the organization must have documentation in the patient record to support the codes assigned. Therefore, the physician may be required to add an addendum or additional note to the medical record to provide clarification of his or her documentation. The AHIMA Practice Brief provides guidance on query content, wording, and use.

Finally, each organization should consider establishing the query as part of the record so that it can be tracked and the physician can be sanctioned for failure to respond to queries in a timely manner.

Coding summary

Utilizing the functionality of the encoder, a coding summary document should be placed within the patient record. The summary will be kept as a permanent part of the patient record. The benefit of capturing the coding summary in the record includes providing a source document for auditors when they are assessing the accuracy of the coding performed by coders, to compare to codes that appear on the claim and identify discrepancies between codes submitted for claim purposes versus codes appearing on the claim, and to serve as a document type in the electronic health record that provides an index of conditions for which the patient was treated and can be quickly accessed by caregivers.

Data quality and integrity

Consistent with AHIMA's *Standards of Ethical Coding*, all coding staff:

- Will not misrepresent services that were rendered in order to optimize reimbursement or for any other reason.
- Will report any variances from the coding compliance plan to the coding manager, director of health information management, or the organization's compliance officer or hotline.
- Will avoid applying codes to cases that are outside of their level of coding expertise, unless the coding is validated by a coworker or supervisor with the expertise.
- Will answer physician office's and patient financial service's coding questions, within the level of their expertise; collaborate with their colleagues on cases with complex coding requirements; and assist in updating superbills, charge sheets, encounter forms, and the charge description master (CDM), within the level of their coding expertise.
- Will not add diagnosis codes based solely on test results.
- Will not report diagnoses and procedures that the physician has specifically indicated he or she does not support.
- Will query the physician when documentation is unclear, is ambiguous, conflicts with test results, or does not support medical necessity of services provided.

- Will not deviate from official coding guidelines in order to get a claim paid unless unique payer requirements are received in writing.

- Will further develop their skill and knowledge of coding and classification systems and official resources in order to select the appropriate diagnostic and procedural codes.

- Will participate in the development of institutional coding policies and ensure policies do not conflict with official coding rules and guidelines.

The organization may wish to include expectations for providers (especially when the physician or nonphysician provider applies codes that transfer directly to claims without being reviewed by a certified coder) and patient financial services and access (or registration) in this policy. Examples of components that may be appropriate appear in the book *JustCoding's Practical Guide to Coding Management.*

Coding compliance subcommittee

ABC's coding compliance subcommittee conducts coding compliance activities and reports its activities, planned audits, and findings to the compliance committee. The duties of the subcommittee include:

- Monitoring compliance with this plan and reporting noncompliance to the compliance officer

- Evaluating and recommending training and education needs of staff with regard to coding, reimbursement, and documentation compliance issues

- Implementing the audit schedule

- Evaluating and updating existing policies, procedures, and processes that relate to coding and reimbursement compliance and developing policies and procedures for issues or processes not addressed in existing policies and procedures

- Evaluating the existing and/or recommending needed equipment and technology solutions to support and improve coding, physician documentation, and reimbursement
- Assessing the impact and resource requirements of new legislation and regulatory requirements upon coding, billing, and physician documentation and making resource and process recommendations as appropriate

Hopefully, the outline above provided sufficient content to assist you in developing your coding compliance plan. As mentioned earlier, the plan is dynamic, and one can see several components mentioned above that could change in the future, including the impending coding classification system ICD-11.

What Should Be Audited

Managers should not assume that they can review every coding guideline, *Coding Clinic*, or coding-related issue targeted by the Office of Inspector General (OIG) or RAC; thus, frequent audits are important. The coding manager, lead coder, and coding auditor's responsibilities include:

- Planning the coding audit process
- Organizing the resources necessary to conduct these audits, which will assess the coding staff's skills
- Encouraging staff members to learn more about disease processes and clinical interventions to improve their coding performance

An internal coding audit program is the monitoring effort that ties together all coding management functions. Audit topics must be significant to the organization, monitor changes in coding practice, address claim rejection or denial reasons, and provide an opportunity for each coder (and provider's coding) to be assessed.

When determining what topics to audit, one goal should be to improve the coding team's performance. Managers should consider whether any of their coders are new to the profession or team. Managers could monitor their performance to determine whether it is at an appropriate level. Coding quality is typically expected to be at 95%, according to the 2017 HCPro coding benchmark survey. Managers must determine whether any new coders are meeting this level of proficiency. Conducting an audit of their current work can answer that question and lend insight regarding necessary corrective measures. Remember that corrective measures are not intended to be punitive actions but rather actions that improve performance, which may include focused education, additional reference materials, or closer monitoring.

Similarly, if your physicians and nonphysician providers are applying codes that transfer directly to the claim without any review, the coding performed by these clinicians should be reviewed. If they are new to your organization, then initially monitoring a large sample of their work may be appropriate. Documentation, coding practices and rules, and query response expectations should be part of a new clinician's orientation to the organization and serve as the basis for reporting for recredentialing purposes, record delinquencies, and other quality measures. Below is an excerpt of a physician coding compliance plan that may assist you in determining what to include in yours (see Fig. 4.2).

FIGURE 4.2 PRACTITIONER CODING COMPLIANCE PLAN

Any new practitioner (either employed or contracted) is required to attend an introductory training course in E/M, modifier, and procedural coding provided by the coding compliance counselor within two weeks of beginning work. This training is required for ALL practitioners (physicians and APPs), regardless of their prior experience and coding training.

ALL practitioners are required to attend a minimum of one coding update training course, annually, including the definitions and use of modifiers that support services provided. This requirement will help practitioners learn all new coding guidelines and reinforce key existing coding concepts. This course will be arranged and provided by ABC's coding compliance counselor.

Practitioners will receive feedback and training as part of their annual E/M coding review. See further discussion in the "Audits" section below. They also will receive feedback and guidance from the coding compliance counselor and the practice's billing service throughout the year as coders review their procedural codes and modifier use. Periodically, the coding compliance counselor will be on-site at practices and available for practitioners' questions and to observe how practitioners are coding and provide feedback

The coding compliance counselor is responsible for determining the content and extent of training required within the guidelines described herein for both staff and practitioners, in consultation with the HIM director, billing service director, practice manager, and the chief medical officer.

Audits
Coding reviews will be performed as follows:

- 50% of new practitioner procedural and E/M codes submitted are reviewed by the coding compliance counselor for 60 days.

- Annually, an independent company will perform an audit of diagnosis, procedural, and E/M codes, including appropriate use of modifiers. This is meant to be an overall compliance audit to independently confirm that the plan is effective.

- Annually, on or near the practitioner's hire date anniversary, a review of the practitioner's coding will be conducted. Appropriate modifier use will be audited in addition to the E/M, CPT, and diagnosis code review. This review will be conducted by the coding compliance counselor.

  o A sample of 20 encounters per practitioner will be audited from the most recent 60 days of service for each practitioner. Random charts will be selected by the coding compliance counselor to audit based on a number of factors, including, but not limited to, risk areas identified by the Office of Inspector General, or other regulatory agencies, new coding regulations, and history of past coding errors or denials either by the specific practitioner being audited or other practitioners within the practice.

FIGURE 4.2 PRACTITIONER CODING COMPLIANCE PLAN (CONT.)

- The coding compliance counselor will discuss the results of the review with the practitioner to allow the practitioner to clarify or provide additional information to support coding that may be identified initially as inaccurate. The coding compliance counselor will provide education relative to coding errors and update information, where applicable. The practice manager and a representative from the Compliance Department shall be present at these meetings. A representative from the billing service may attend.

- Practitioners are expected to achieve and maintain a coding accuracy rate of 90% or higher for E/M, CPT, and diagnoses. Although the use of appropriate modifiers is ultimately the responsibility of the practitioner, the audited results for modifiers will be documented for training and review but will not be included in the overall score. Scoring criteria shall be utilized and shared with the practitioner in advance. If a practitioner does not pass his or her audit, the following escalation process will occur:

  o The practitioner will receive education on the area(s) where the expectation was not achieved.

  o Each of the practitioner's encounters will be placed on "billing hold" until the coding compliance counselor or other contracted individual is able to assess the accuracy of the practitioner's coding. Feedback will be provided to the practitioner at least weekly.

    – If this is the first occurrence of coding accuracy falling below 90%, there will be no impact to the practitioner's compensation plan. If this is a subsequent occurrence, the practitioner's compensation plan will be adjusted by the cost of staff conducting the reviews.

  o Once the practitioner's coding accuracy achieves and maintains 90% or higher for two or more consecutive weeks, the daily reviews will be stopped.

- The practitioner will be reaudited in approximately 90 days after achieving the 90% level. If a practitioner fails a second review within a 24-month period, the practice manager, as well as the chief medical office and corporate compliance officer, will attend a meeting with the coding compliance counselor and practitioner to review the audit findings and prepare a corrective action plan to be signed by the practitioner. This plan shall include a follow-up education session with the coding compliance counselor and daily reviews of encounters on hold as described earlier. On this occurrence, the practitioner shall incur the cost of the daily reviews.

- Copies of audit reports shall be distributed to the coding manager, chief medical officer, compliance officer, and practice manager as appropriate. A summary of review results will be provided to corporate compliance quarterly.

- A master set of all coding results shall be maintained by the coding compliance counselor.

- The coding compliance counselor will report to the billing service those accounts that require rebilling as a result of the reviews.

Source: Rose T. Dunn. Reprinted with permission.

When one is creating a coding compliance plan for the professional staff, it is important to involve the chief medical officer or president of the medical and professional staff as well as a provider or two to provide input. You may find that they have topics they wish to have reviewed and from which they can gain some additional education. Having these individuals involved will assist you in discussing the program with others on the medical and professional staff, and these collaborators will help "sell" the program to their colleagues.

Other Sources of Review Topics

External or internal audits that have identified weaknesses and claim denials attributable to coding may signal other areas to monitor. Capturing denial reasons attributable to coding errors helps to identify the ideal topics to use for in-services. Managers can use the findings to implement education programs that can help reduce denials. Reducing coding denials is something tangible to demonstrate the value of your team members to upper management. Managers also may consider auditing confusing conditions, such as modifier -25, incident-to requirements, sepsis, and septicemia, or documentation-driven services, such as infusions for which the combination of inadequate documentation of start and stop times and improper coding yields less revenue than the organization anticipated.

Limit reviews

Managers confronted with multiple appropriate issues to monitor should focus on one at a time until each is resolved and team members are performing at the level expected of them. Internal reviews should apply to all team members, including contractors, and all activities that the team members perform. If team members abstract data into the computer system, periodically review that abstracted data for accuracy. Review discharge dispositions if coders validate them. With many options of topics to monitor, managers should consider developing an internal audit calendar to help stay on track. Share this calendar with the team members and the compliance department so everyone is aware of each month's focus.

FIGURE 4.3 CODING COMPLIANCE CALENDAR

ABC Medical Center coding compliance calendar	
The reviews appearing in this calendar will apply to all employed practitioners and all employed and contracted coders.	
JANUARY: Coder and practitioner education on new CPT-4 codes, new CPT-4 codes audits, CDI mismatches	**FEBRUARY:** HCC claim comparison to prior year for missing HCCs
MARCH: DRG CC/MCC capture for inpatient records; CDI mismatches	**APRIL:** POA and discharge disposition review, CDI mismatches, common denial conditions review
MAY: Recredentialing reviews of all practitioners	**JUNE:** Modifier usage for outpatient surgery and ED coding, ED facility leveling, ED ProFee coding
JULY: New practitioner coding education, coding reviews, teaching supervision documentation	**AUGUST:** Random review of each coder's cases, CDI mismatches
SEPTEMBER: Chemotherapy, observation, and clinic encounters (including ProFee codes), OIG *Work Plan* topics	**OCTOBER:** Education on new ICD-10-CM/PCS codes, new code usage review, CDI mismatches
NOVEMBER: Contracted inpatient, outpatient, and ProFee review	**DECEMBER:** CMI analysis, common denial conditions review

Source: Rose T. Dunn. Reprinted with permission.

While much content has been provided for your development of a coding compliance plan and program, there are other components you should consider incorporating in the plan.

Examples of additional content for the coding compliance plan

Coding audit sample and frequency

Internal reviews for new coders:

- 100% of the cases coded by a newly employed, experienced, and certified/credentialed coder will be reviewed for the first two weeks. If the coder's accuracy is not at least 95% at the end of the two-week period, the reviews will continue. If the newly hired coder is at 95% at the end of the two-week period, the frequency of reviews will be in accordance with the coding compliance plan.
- 100% of all cases coded by a noncertified/noncredentialed, nonexperienced, newly employed coder will be reviewed until such time that the coder achieves a 95% accuracy rating for two consecutive weeks or 60 consecutive cases, whichever criterion achieves a larger sample.

External reviews for coders in their first year of employment or coders who have not achieved 95% accuracy:

- Inpatient coding: Quarterly. Thirty randomly selected discharges for each coder coding inpatient stays.
- Outpatient coding: Quarterly. Thirty randomly selected noninvasive encounters for each coder coding noninvasive services. Forty randomly selected invasive encounters for each coder coding invasive services.
- ProFee coding: Quarterly. Sixty randomly selected encounters, with no less than 20 being inpatient encounters for each coder coding ProFee services.
- Audit focus should include the accuracy of:
    - Diagnosis coding (capture and code assignment)
    - Present on admission
    - Procedure coding (CPT or ICD-10-PCS)
    - Sequencing

- Diagnosis-related groups (DRG) and ambulatory payment classifications (APC)
- E/M levels
- Facility levels
- Disposition
- Query content and use

External reviews conducted for coders in their second year and thereafter are the same as above but on a semiannual frequency.

Internal reviews should happen each month, and the coding manager will review four randomly selected cases for each coder with the same components of the audit focus above.

Coding accuracy rate will be calculated using the code-over-code methodology. Reimbursement accuracy rate will be based on the accuracy of the DRGs and APCs derived using the case-over-case methodology.

Audit focus

Consider all options that may be available, as well as the audit calendar. Below are several areas of focus to consider:

- Data transfer: Review of the patient record to determine accurate code assignment with subsequent comparison with the appropriate claim form (UB-04, CMS 1500, etc.) to confirm codes are properly transferring to the claim. This is a way to determine whether hard codes from the CDM are duplicating soft codes that were applied by the coders.
- Regulatory issues: Focus areas should include issues noted in or by the current OIG *Work Plan*, RAC, Medicaid Integrity Contractor, and any specific payer (e.g., Medicare Advantage). Consider partnering with patient financial services to validate other codes on the claim, such as

place of service (see OIG audit report 11300506 from May 2015 that identified substantial overpayments for this coding error).

- Documentation integrity issues: Properly authenticated entries, abbreviation usage, copy-forward frequency and appropriateness, ongoing record review findings, etc. We have discussed some of these relative to the RADV audits. However, the *Program Integrity Manual*, CMS Pub 100-08 §3.3.2.4, has signature requirements as well. If the signature is missing from an order, MACs and CERT will disregard the order during the review of the claim (e.g., the reviewer will proceed as if the order was not received). This means that if a service was rendered and billed for based on the unauthenticated order, we have a revenue integrity issue. If the signature is missing from any other medical documentation (other than an order), MACs and CERT may accept a signature attestation from the author of the medical record entry.

Remember, the findings from our reviews should be utilized to improve coding and patient record documentation practices and to identify educational opportunities for coders, practitioners, and clinical documentation improvement specialists. As for the latter, the coding compliance program may consider establishing a standing educational meeting, perhaps on a quarterly basis. The findings from the reviews of the prior quarter will serve to identify the topics to be discussed, the intended audience, and whether external speakers may need to be engaged to deliver the program.

Protecting the Findings

The coding compliance plan should speak to whether the audits that are conducted, both internally and by contracted external agents, are to be performed under an attorney privilege umbrella. This approach may be appropriate if you know you have or anticipate finding significant coding and billing problems. While the guidance below refers to hospitals, it is applicable to skilled nursing facilities, outpatient facilities, and physician practices as well.

FIGURE 4.4

Coding audits and attorney-client privilege

If your facility uncovers a problematic coding and billing problem, it may be appropriate to consult an outside attorney. The attorney-client privilege has significant historical roots. Generally, the privilege protects communications between an attorney and his or her client. The terms "attorney" and "client" are important in the application of the privilege. In a 1981 case, the court noted that the privilege protects from disclosure communications that are all of the following:

1. Received in confidence

2. Between a client and an attorney

3. For purposes of obtaining legal advice

Application of the attorney-client privilege is determined on a case-by-case basis. This makes the privilege itself somewhat tenuous. The safest way to preserve the attorney-client privilege is to engage outside counsel adhering to specific preestablished guidelines. The hospital must be willing to abide by the limitations and standards the attorney places on the relationship. Management must implicitly understand how the attorney-client relationship will alter the hospital's behavior. The hospital must accept the legal, operational, and economic ramifications of the attorney-client relationship designed to protect audit findings.

If the attorney-client privilege protection is going to be successful in court, the hospital must do the following:

1. Delegate control to outside counsel. The hospital may only share audit information with very limited parties (usually top-level managers). Furthermore, audit results may not be shared with the HIM department for feedback and comments. All communications regarding the audit must be funneled through the attorney. The hospital should not communicate with the audit firm directly. These are just some constraints of the relationship. The bottom line is that the hospital must give up most of its control over the audit process and entrust a great deal to the outside law firm.

FIGURE 4.4 (CONT.)

---

2. Implicitly trust the competency of both the law firm and the audit firm. To do this, hospitals should be sure to retain outside counsel with experience in attorney-client privileged audits and healthcare reimbursement audits. The audit firm should also have experience with attorney-client privileged situations. This is a highly sensitive area and should not be one that the hospital leaves open to chance, even if it means not dealing with the same law firm or audit firm the organization has depended on for a decade.

3. Determine whether the added expense is worth the added protection. You cannot put a price tag on the legal protection the law firm may bring to your audit process, but you still need to be prepared for the additional expense. The hospital should perform a cost-benefit analysis so that it can justify its decision to retain or not retain outside counsel. In the end, the hospital's decision must rest on both the legal and compliance competency of the law firm, as well as the law firm's experience with reimbursement audits.

Source: HCPro.

If the review is a routine review with no anticipated significant issues, then routine handling of the findings should occur with distribution primarily to the compliance officer. The compliance officer is the organization's point person for all compliance activities, including coding audits. As a result of the audit findings, the compliance officer must determine whether refunds should be made to payers.

According to Richard L. Bouma, author of "Medicare's 60-Day Overpayment Rule: Uncorrected Mistakes Become False Claims" (2012), "Medicare requires the provider to proactively return the money. Specifically, under the 2010 Affordable Care Act, a Medicare provider has an obligation to return that reimbursement to Medicare within 60 days after the overpayment has been 'identified.' If the provider fails to meet that 60-day deadline, the provider becomes liable for substantial penalties under the False Claims Act and also risks exclusion from the Medicare program."

This guidance was further clarified by CMS on March 14, 2016 (emphasis added):

*Overpayments must be returned either within 60 days of being identi-fied **or by the date the corresponding cost report (applicable to pay-ments to hospitals) is due, whichever is later.** Overpayments must be reported and returned if identified within 6 years of the overpayment being received.*

The compliance officer recognizes the CMS timetable discussed above and will collaborate with the HIM director, coding manager, coding compliance auditor, and patient financial services regarding any rebilling and/or refund activities and assess the need for further compliance-related actions.

Summary

Every organization should have a coding compliance policy and plan. Develop-ing the plan will take time to consider the who, what, when, and how compo-nents of the compliance program. Implementation will take some planning, and a coding auditing calendar may assist in organizing the auditing efforts and ensuring sufficient resources are available to complete the tasks. Extending the reviews to areas other than coding may be beneficial for the organization and can be done in collaboration with the coding compliance auditor's activ-ities. Regardless of what may or may not be known when coding audits are conducted, it may be beneficial to involve legal counsel. Recognizing the CMS ruling regarding refunding overpayments is one factor that must be kept in mind once the audit findings are reported. Next, we will review some of the issues that payers investigate in their audit activities.

REFERENCES

AHIMA. 2016. "Guidelines for Achieving a Compliant Query Practice (2016 Update)". Retrieved from *http://library.ahima.org/PB/QueryCompliance#.Wk1KzN8m5Jk*.

Bouma, R. L. 2012. "Medicare's 60-Day Overpayment Rule: Uncorrected Mistakes Become False Claims." Warner, Norcross & Judd. Retrieved from *https://www.wnj.com/Publications/ Medicare%E2%80%99s-60-Day-Overpayment-Rule-Uncorrected-Mis*.

CMS. 2012. "Recovery Audit Program Diagnosis Related Group (DRG) Coding Vulnerabilities for Inpatient Hospitals Accessed." Retrieved from *https://www.cms.gov/Outreach-and-Education/ Medicare-Learning-Network-MLN/MLNMattersArticles/downloads/se1121.pdf*.

CMS. 2016. "Medicare Program; Reporting and Returning of Overpayments." *Federal Register, The Daily Journal of the United States Government*. Retrieved from *https://www.federalregister.gov/ documents/2016/02/12/2016-02789/medicare-program-reporting-and-returning-of-overpayments*.

Dunn, R.T. 2016. JustCoding's Practical Guide to Coding Management. Middleton, MA: HCPro, Inc.

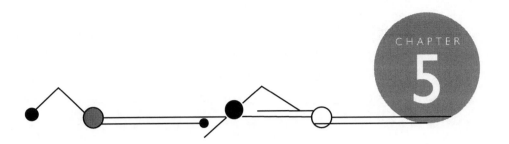

Audit Focus and the Approach of Insurers

CHAPTER OBJECTIVES

- Characterize the types of payer audits
- Discuss the payer's use of data analytics and pattern tracking
- Summarize the documentation elements monitored by payers
- Review issues commonly reviewed by payers
- Understand how the payer's contract may affect their access to your records

Types of Audits

Line item audits

Line item audits are the traditional audit technique of most commercial payers. This type of audit focuses on the charge lines themselves and reconciles the charges with the medical record. The facility/doctor will send the itemized claim of each charge through to the payer, who will reconcile it with the medical record and orders. Items not documented in the record will be disallowed, thereby reducing the total charges.

This type of audit is based on the fee-for-service methodology and has a singular focus of ensuring the payer reimburses only documented services, supplies, and tests. The importance of the line item audit has diminished in recent years with the advent of value- and risk-based contracting but remains a very significant audit type. Auditors for these types of audits are either employed by the payer itself or an independent contractor receiving a portion of the findings by which the total claim was reduced.

HEDIS audits

The Healthcare Effectiveness Data and Information Set (HEDIS) is the responsibility of the National Committee for Quality Assurance (NCQA). The goal of the HEDIS is stated by the NCQA as "devising a standardized set of performance measures that could be used by various constituencies to compare health plans" (NCQA, n.d.).

According to the NCQA, approximately 90% of insurance plans collect and report HEDIS data. The auditor would use the HEDIS audit specifications as published in the technical manual. All the audit guidelines, specifications, and reporting requirements can be found on their website at *www.ncqa.org/hedis-quality-measurement/data-reporting-services/ hedis-compliance-audit-program.*

Most payers either contract with an external firm or utilize internal auditors to specifically address the measures, as required by HEDIS. Ultimately, what they report will reflect on their overall performance when measured against other plans. Therefore, payers place strong significance and resources on the HEDIS audit criteria.

DRG/DRG validation audits

These audits span the breadth of governmental, commercial, and managed care payers. They are an in-depth review of the medical record documentation as reconciled with the coding criteria. Auditors review the inpatient record specifically to validate that the assigned diagnosis-related group (DRG) is documented and should be reimbursed as assigned. Most payers publish an internal document to guide the auditors with the DRG process. One such document is published by Tufts Health Plan and can be found on their website at *www.tuftshealthplan.com/documents/providers/payment-policies/drg-audit-policy*.

Like other audit types, these can be performed within the payer system itself or contracted out. The payers depend upon advanced data analytics to select the DRG for validation and are becoming increasingly successful at downgrading the DRG, resulting in less reimbursement for the facility. Facilities should use the documents on the payer website and perform routine random audits that "mimic" the DRG validation internally to limit their denials and downgrades.

Medical necessity audits

The commercial payer method of determining medical necessity and the government method are both generally based on published criteria. That is where the similarity stops. Commercial payer/managed care audits generally determine some components based on the medical necessity guidelines and prior authorization requirements. In many cases, there is regular interaction between the case managers at the facility and the case manager for the payer. These interactions are documented and audited to ensure the medical necessity for the stay or service is documented and supported by the record; therefore, this is both a concurrent and retrospective form of audit.

This differs from a government audit that is entirely retrospective. Payers may follow Medicare guidelines but are not required to do so unless it is a Medicare Advantage program. Even so, the payer, as a contractor, can amend or supplement some of the medical necessity criteria; therefore, payers will require documentation supportive of the claim, and the payer auditor (internal or contracted) will reconcile against the medical record.

Payers Driven by Financial Results

Insurers are in business to make a profit. This profit comes from the difference between what is paid in premiums and the reimbursement provided. They are the sole entity in the United States allowed to manage "risk," and for taking the risk they set some guidelines to ensure medically necessary services are reimbursed.

Stronger guidelines and limitations will occur around high-dollar costs to the payer, such as chronic disease and mental health services. In order to manage their risk, they rely heavily on the use of data and data analytics. While federal payers do use data analytics, to a large degree they are neophytes compared to the sophistication of the commercial and managed care payers.

Data analytics and claim selection process

Commercial and managed care payers have huge repositories of claim data for which they can use predictive analytics to determine patterns of behavior, which determine the claims within their benchmark. Claims that fall outside the benchmark or demonstrate an aberrant data element will be selected for review. A payer auditor, whether internal or contract, will receive the claim information and the medical record. In addition, the potential concern will be highlighted. This occurs in much the same fashion as the Program for Evaluating Payment Patterns Electronic Report (PEPPER) does for Medicare.

In addition, if the payer audit staff determines there may be a pattern of behavior of inappropriate charges, then more records will be selected. Let's, for example, assume there is a "carveout" in the contract for revenue code 278 implants. The data and the auditor note that there appear to be supplies in this revenue code that would not be eligible for carveout. This is one example of how the claims would be selected. The payer auditor will receive claim review information based on millions of historical claims that can detect outliers in a laser-focused fashion.

This focus is generally applied to high-dollar claims, high-dollar pharmaceuticals, readmissions, chronic diseases, and many more categories.

The role of the selection nurse

Many, but not all, payers and payer contractors still use a second-level selection performed by a selection nurse. This role is becoming obsolete based on the advancement of data analytics using the data scientist. However, if a selection nurse is involved, he or she will review the account for "probability" of an incorrect reimbursement or lack of medical necessity.

The selection nurse will use all the diagnosis codes submitted on the claim to determine whether the codes on the claim or DRG are medically necessary. Selection nurses still excel in areas of high-dollar pharmaceuticals, cancer care, and high-dollar claims such as transplants. The goal of the selection nurse is to select only those claims where there is a likely inappropriate payment by the payer. Once selected, the claim can take several paths, from DRG validation, medical necessity validation, health information management review, and even a line item review of charges. Each claim that is reviewed represents additional costs to the payer; therefore, every effort is made to ensure that only those with potential errors are selected.

The importance of patterns of behavior

Big data analytics uses the "three Vs" to analyze data: volume, velocity, and variety. Many software vendors today offer machine-learning analytics to providers and facilities to capture lost charges and undercharges (SAS, n.d.). In the same fashion, payers enlist data scientists to review millions of pieces of data to determine patterns that are both expected and unexpected. The payer will further review the unexpected patterns and either determine these patterns to be valid, representing an overpayment, or a false positive, which would be removed in future analytics.

A common example of this type of analytics is the PEPPER used to compare hospitals and other providers against peers in their state, jurisdiction, and nation (TMF, n.d.). Payer analytics in many ways do the same thing—compare the facility against itself, its ZIP code, its state, and the entire nation. Similar metrics are created for providers to determine who has the highest-quality outcomes with the least cost. These become the preferred providers. A payer audit group can go through thousands of claims in minutes to detect outliers, giving them a systematic advantage over the provider. Patterns of behavior detected by a payer are not unlike those of Medicare and can rise and fall in charge volume.

It is through the data analytics, selection nurse auditors, and pattern detection that the payers begin the audit process. We will change the focus now to what the payer expects from facilities and providers in terms of documentation to support the claimed service(s).

What Payers Are Looking For

There is a lot of confusion in the industry about what a commercial/managed care payer would want in order to approve the claim. Much of this confusion comes from the timing of requirements to ensure reimbursement. The bottom line is the same for all payers: The documentation must show a plan of care based on the working diagnosis and then progress to the goal of the plan and when the patient can expect to reach the goal. One documentation system should be characteristic of each provider or facility, and it should not display wide variations within the same provider identification and documentation methods. Electronic medical records (EMR) have complicated the documentation process with the inclusion of thousands of nonessential elements for the sole purpose of data collection and not for the support of the care provided. Despite variations in documentation, the following elements are critical to supportive documentation.

Payer guideline compliance

Medicare provides guidance through national and local coverage determinations—articles that set forth the standards that must be followed to attain a benefit category and reimbursement. Similarly, each payer provides its own guidelines based on their management of "risk." While many follow Medicare guidelines, they can certainly produce their own guidelines per their contracts. Payer guidelines generally address items such as:

- Medical necessity
- Prior authorization requirements
- Preadmission guidelines
- Therapy requirement
- Formulary and nonformulary medications
- Other requirements based on payer operations

Additional payer guidance may be included within the contract with the payer. Many payers publish their guidelines in either hard copy or through their websites. All guidelines are proprietary to the payer; therefore, a facility or provider cannot apply these as "universal" guidelines for all payers. An example of a payer guideline is the joint arthroplasty guideline published by BlueCross of Florida. This example can be found on the BlueCross website at *mcgs.bcbsfl. com/?doc=Knee%20Arthroplasty.*

Within this document, there is an overview followed by the criteria that must be met for authorization for the procedure and aftercare. The payer auditor will take this guideline and review each component against the medical record documentation to see that the criteria have been achieved. Failure to follow these guidelines will most likely result in a denial of the claim. It is important to note that this guideline would only specifically apply to BlueCross but may in fact be similar to other payer's guidelines for the same procedure. If a facility performs a significant number of arthroplasties, then the creation of a documentation template against the guidelines would be one method to ensure compliance with the payer-stated guidelines.

Payer guidelines, like Medicare, are dynamic and subject to change at any time. Therefore, the documentation in the record must support the guideline in existence on the day the service was rendered. Like national and local coverage determinations for Medicare, these are expected to be well documented within the medical record and address each element of the guideline completely. Every provider should randomly audit their record against the relevant payer guidelines to ensure that the record is complete and addresses the guidelines.

Medical necessity compliance

Like payer guidance, medical necessity must be met and documented prior to claim submission. Sometimes the medical necessity requirements are listed within the payer guidelines, and other times they may be in a separate document. Medical necessity requirements quite often are similar to those required for Medicare. The bottom line is that a payer will expect to see the outpatient need for the service or the inpatient plan of care. To this extent, they may follow various screening tools, but these are not the only requirements that need to be satisfied for a payer. In most cases, there needs to be a fully developed active problem list showing the plan of care to address the active problems. There is also an expectation that within the plan there are regular updates on progress toward the stated goal or evidence that the plan was changed to adjust the goal. Payers use many different medical necessity formats. For example, there are substantial medical necessity guidelines surrounding chronic care conditions, such as behavioral health.

Magellan publishes their documentation requirements specific to each type of service whether inpatient, intensive outpatient, or partial hospitalization

(Magellan Healthcare, 2016). For many chronic conditions, as well as acute conditions, there will be guidelines that specify what must be documented to achieve medical necessity. Unlike Medicare, most commercial or managed care payers require medical necessity determination early in the episode of care in order to provide further authorization for the service. A payer will therefore want to see all case management notes documenting their review of the plan of care, progress as stated by the provider, and discussions they have had with the payer case management. Failure of the provider or facility to engage with the appropriate case management at the payer level will put the claim in jeopardy for reimbursement, as medical necessity is dynamic and must be reassessed at each step of the care plan. This is different from Medicare where all medical necessity is performed retrospectively. If at any point medical necessity is not achieved, then the service is deemed to be complete; therefore, it is essential that screening tools be used throughout the stay and specific documentation by the case management be in place to document communication with the payer on the plan of care and expectation for length of stay.

Arguably, documentation requirements for commercial or managed care payers, in terms of medical necessity, can be more extensive than for Medicare. With the growth in commercial/managed care and Medicaid plans, it is essential that documentation now be based on these growing percentages of the payer mix instead of solely on Medicare. Payers will also need to see evidence that the beneficiary is in the most appropriate location and status to receive the medically necessary care with the highest-quality outcome and lowest cost. Therefore, like Medicare status, evaluations are common in medical necessity determination processes.

Documentation of services rendered as necessary

This element is of particular importance and required by all commercial/managed care payers, as they may use a charge line audit. Every test, service, procedure, pharmaceutical, and nonroutine supply must have an order and be clearly documented within the record. The auditor will compare the itemized claim data (not the UB04 or CMS 1500) of charges and reconcile every line to the medical record. If there is not complete documentation, the service will be determined as not documented and removed from the total charges to be reimbursed. This process applies to both inpatient and outpatient services.

Overutilization of testing is also reviewed against payer guidelines and evidence-based medicine guidelines. As such, "routine" tests ordered each day that are not directly related to the plan of care become a potential for removal from the charges. Pharmaceuticals are of particular importance in the payers' review. Pharmaceuticals are either formulary or nonformulary and audited as such. Some tests and medications require that a more conservative treatment has been tried and failed prior to moving on to a more expensive pharmacy or treatment.

This is especially important with high-cost drugs. A payer will expect to see that the provider has considered a more generic or lower-cost alternative and documented why it was not in the interest of the beneficiary to have had that medication. In some cases, the payer will issue payer guidelines that include medical necessity requirements for medications. Payer data analytics are sophisticated, and these claims are targeted more for review, so documentation that the services/medications are necessary is an expectation of the payer.

Avoidance of nonessential overutilization of testing

As mentioned previously, facilities seek to avoid litigation and document care through testing. However, if the provider does not speak to the value of the testing as an element of the plan of care, then it can be deemed routine or nonessential, such as "daily labs" that are not discussed in the progress note or shown in the documentation of medical decision-making. This can result in a determination of non–medically necessary testing. With the advent of value-based care and "risk sharing" contracts, overutilization has come into focus for both the provider and payer. In some cases, joint utilization programs have been developed. One example is the Cleveland Clinic Test Utilization program. These programs are geared, as are payer programs, at the reduction of overutilization of testing.

As providers are moving toward value and away from fee-for-service, the focus on reducing overutilization by payers becomes significant. Furthermore, the advent of downside risk sharing arrangements puts overutilization at top of the auditors' minds and comes into focus in the line item audit. Facilities should conduct ongoing line item internal audits to determine whether they have concerns with overutilization. As we move to a downside risk payer-provider model, one key goal will be reduction in the cost to provide care. Therefore, payer auditors will be focused on this goal.

Delay of care events

One consistent focus of governmental and commercial/managed care payer over time has been charges that resulted from a delay of care. Therefore, most payers perform routine audits of high-dollar or high-volume admissions over a weekend and holiday to determine whether the patient received care in a timely fashion and met that medically necessary inpatient level of care. It is important to note that most commercial/managed care admissions require notification of the payer and then ongoing case manager–to–case manager discussions. Most of the potential delay-of-care concerns will be addressed at this point.

However, auditors will look to see that the documentation for the medical plan of care and necessary testing shows a reasonable time frame and has not been delayed. For example, a patient is admitted for chest pain on a Thursday, and the plan of care calls for a diagnostic cardiac catheterization and stress test. However, the record sees the orders marked as urgent, but it is electively scheduled for the following Tuesday, when Dr. Smith comes back to town.

This would be an example where care was delayed for a selected physician and would likely result in a denial. Delay-of-care issues are less likely with commercial/managed care payers who have ongoing case management discussions during the patients' hospital stay than with the federal payers who are not prospective but retrospective in their audit methods. Having said that, all payers still focus on delay of services within their audit techniques. The plan of care, severity of illness, and receiving care must be efficiently provided and recorded in the medical record.

Never events

Most commercial/managed care payers follow the Agency for Healthcare Research and Quality (AHRQ) never event guidelines. Nonfederal payers generally will not provide reimbursement for a never event or care required to remedy the malady created by the never event. Never events came into the commercial payer arena in 2008, and most payers outline their management of these events within the payer-provider contract or within the benefit manuals published by the payer.

In 2008, Healthcare Finance published the concerns that Cigna had with never events and reimbursement for these events (Healthcare Finance, 2008). Most payers require the provider (whether physician or facility) to report a never event to them within a specified amount of time after the event occurs. When reported, the payer has a guideline for auditing and continued monitoring of the patient claims and medical record. Some states supersede payer requirements and require a root cause analysis and report of remediation be issued. The payer, at a minimum, will be requesting the full medical record for an indeterminate amount of time into the future to ensure they are not reimbursing for the never event.

Payer Audit Characteristic Summary

Payer audits are generally based on sophisticated data analytics and predictive analytics (including machine learning). Facilities, however, seldom perform routine random audits prior to claim selection. This disparity allows the payer to benefit from detectable patterns of behavior that then result in targeted audits.

Once the selection occurs, additional data analytics help to identify concerns within the claim. The payer will expect complete medical records, and this can be difficult, as some EMRs do not print the entire record as seen on the screen or print such a volume of nonrequired data that it is overwhelming to the payer auditor. The payer will expect a record that is complete in documentation, demonstrating a plan of care, progress, and/or achievement of the goal of the plan. Additionally, they will be looking for nonessential testing or testing the provider does not include in the medical decision-making notes.

In many cases, a commercial/managed care payer will have higher expectations than a Medicare contractor. However, the level of documentation required with line item audits is extensive so that complete reconciliation of the claim to the medical record exists. It is incumbent on the facility to have printed and reviewed the record prior to submitting as part of an automated data request. Failure to include all necessary documentation may cause a technical denial of reimbursement.

Payer contract affects the request and review

Unlike federal and state payers, commercial/managed care and even accountable care organizations (ACO) will have very specific language in the contracts regarding reimbursement. These contracts may actually alter or fail to accept Medicare or Medicaid guidelines. In the case of a commercial/managed care payer, the key to successful implementation of contract guidelines is to formulate a facility or provider-based team. This team should always include contract management, case management, utilization management, and someone from the information technology department that will ensure that specific documentation requirements of the contracts are included in all necessary templates.

When it comes to a commercial/managed care payer, their auditors receive the guidelines but generally not the contract signed between the facility and the payer. Therefore, the responsibility for ensuring accurate decisions optimal to the facility will need to come from the facility. Auditors are using guidelines, but there may be some alterations to these specifically stated in the contract. In such a case, the facility can redirect the auditor and prevent a denial. Contracts specifically state any carveout or stop-loss provisions. This is also key to ensuring correct reimbursement. Every facility should create "contract cards" or "scorecards" that state the payer, any specific reimbursement terms, and any exclusions. These should be shared with all relevant parties within the facility but specifically case management, utilization management, and a physician advisor who will be providing ongoing management of the patient.

Additionally, many of these contracts define the network. Recently, beneficiaries have been struggling with the fact that hospitals are in-network but many of their providers are out of network; therefore, patients have been receiving "surprise bills." Many states have enacted laws against this, but in others even hospitalists are deemed out of network. One aspect that facilities are not as used to communicating is the fact they utilize out-of-network services. The payer knows who is in their network and who is out of network and will pay accordingly. It is incumbent upon the hospital to keep a current list of which providers are in what network, especially if they are employed physicians. This will need to be communicated to the patient so that if possible they can elect the correct providers. Again, the network is defined within the contract.

Line item reviews

We have talked previously about line item reviews. These can occur for either an inpatient or an outpatient. The key to these reviews is that the payer will want to see medical necessity, physician orders, and complete documentation within the medical record.

Let's take normal saline (NS) for an example. The order reads NS at 100 cc/hour for 24 hours. That would be a total of 2,400 cc or roughly two or three 1,000-cc bags of saline on the claim. However, the actual detailed claim has charges for eight bags of 1,000 cc NS. In this case, the auditor will remove five of those bags from the total charges, as the order was specific to the amount to be infused. While this seems rather picky, the charges associated with a review such as this can become extensive. By removing charges from the claim, the total charges will be reduced. Therefore, the payer will pay only the percent of adjusted charges.

Additionally, with high-cost drugs especially, they may lower the total charges to be below stop loss or alter the carveout amount to be less. Therefore, this type of payer audit remains a mainstay methodology among the commercial and managed care payers. Medications are frequent offenders in this type of audit. The payer will take the dispensed amount and convert to the charge units. However, many facilities still struggle with putting the correct number of units on the claim. This is also evident through many of the Medicare Recovery Auditor Contractor (RAC) findings. A payer auditor will review the medications very closely and remove charges for errors in unit calculation, and failure to document medical necessity through the appropriate payer guidance or from an order that is incomplete (such as an order without cosignature) will be denied. This is one area where there are private niche audit firms that work on contingency for a payer. As such, they are meticulous in the removal of overcharges based on documentation. Facilities must remember that when a claim is sent in for reimbursement, they have in fact denoted that all necessary documentation to support the claim is present. Therefore, any claim at any time becomes an audit risk, and with the advent of sophisticated predictive analytics at the payer, the facility could be at risk.

Another area that is frequently reviewed, in the line item auditing, is the CPT/HCPCS code assigned in specific ranges of CPT/HCPCS. Generally, all radiology, laboratory, and most of the medical CPT codes, which are assigned by a charge master, are a target for audit. Payers know that chargemasters are frequently outdated and/or assign improper units of services. This is especially true for services rendered close to January 1, when the codes are updated. All the code-related concerns are easily picked up through analytics during the download of the claim to the payer. In summation, payers have sophisticated analytics that far surpass the facility, allowing them to select claims and target them for line item removal, thereby either denying the whole claim or decreasing the total billed charges.

Whose guidance are they using?

All too often we hear "payers follow Medicare guidelines," but do the nonfederal payers really follow Medicare? The short answer is probably not. Commercial and managed care payers, even Medicare Advantage plans, have flexibility in how they implement guidelines for payment. Most contracts between payer and facility are notoriously silent on this matter. Some legal analysts would state that if it is silent in the contract, then they default to Medicare, but as a matter of rule, this generally does not hold up during litigation. If the facility can get language into the agreed-upon contract that the payer will follow all Medicare guidelines, then that would make the process clearer. Having said that, this type of language is generally rejected by a payer, so that they can control the "risk" of their contract holders.

Back to our question—whose guidance are they using? It's generally a mixture of the Medicare guidelines as well as specific changes based on their printed guidelines. Most payers, but not all, have a website or portal dedicated to their guidelines, payment policies, and medical necessity policies, and some even publish their audit manuals. It is incumbent upon the provider and/or facility to have a library of these documents to ensure when reviewing a claim that has been returned or denied that the appeal would contain a response to the payer guideline, not Medicare's.

We have discussed how a payer behaves, how they select claims, and even how they audit them. We will now shift our focus to creating the best possible documentation that will withstand payer scrutiny.

Understanding the Reviewer Perception

Despite the concerns brought forward about RAC and payer reviews, the majority of reviews by the payers are very accurate. Like most business transactions, there could be different points of view leading to separate conclusions, but most payer auditors follow a prescribed process and guideline.

Most of the auditors hold certifications such as CMAS (certified medical audit specialist) or a coding certification that ensures they follow appropriate methods for record review. Understanding the reviewer perception will assist the reader and providers to ensure the claim and documentation they submit are complete and meet the requirements of the payer.

Since auditing is a science, most payer auditors (especially the contract auditors) follow the audit process with the following steps:

- Identify the purpose and focus of the audit
- Use credible sources and authority to set the standard
- Collect relevant data, or results could be skewed
- Analyze the data by using metrics and statistical methodology along with objective written notes in the medical record
- Determine the findings, prepare the audit report, and recommend change

These steps are standard throughout the audit industry, with little variation, be it a financial, healthcare, defense, or other audit. Key elements are setting the standard using criteria that are relevant and measurable. For example, a payer audit of hip replacement would use the payer guidelines and documentation requirements set forth in the guidelines. They would generally not use Medicaid or other commercial payer but their own guidelines, policies, and memorandums.

Additionally, step three, collecting necessary data, is essential. The auditor should not be collecting data that is not directly relevant to their stated audit focus. For example, if a payer wants to review an inpatient record from January 1, 2017, through January 4, 2017, the data used for the analysis should not include the September 20, 2017, inpatient admission.

Finally, findings are very important. Auditors will record the principal issues with the medical record, but they might also find tangential findings that would help the provider avoid claim submission delays and/or denials. In many institutions, a payer auditor will come on-site to review the record. While the auditor will conduct the review independent of facility or management presence, they frequently will discuss their findings while on-site. Every provider should take full advantage of this opportunity. We will now review some of the special circumstances that a commercial/managed care payer may require.

Special Circumstance Requirements

Requested versus received information

When a request for data comes from the payer, the facility is obligated to send in the requested data according to the time frame specified within the request letter or within their contract. Failure to send the required data will most often result in a denial.

For this reason, every request for data should be treated as if it were a denial, and all internal denial policies/procedures that the facility has created should be followed. As a general rule, the payer will request "all medical documentation" to support a claim. While the medical record may be sent to the payer, the payer auditor may struggle to find the necessary data. With the advent of EMRs, this has become even worse, with the auditor having to go through hundreds of pages that look different from facility to facility. A payer auditor will always appreciate a cover letter specifying the pages the information can be found on.

Let's use a major joint replacement as an example. Let's say that the payer has a policy that they want to see all records that demonstrate that the patient required the replacement. However, the letter does not go into any more specificity. It would be incumbent upon the facility to provide any and all records that are specified within the payer guideline; therefore, the payer auditor would expect to see all physician office notes, all physical therapy/occupational therapy notes (from any location), all medications prescribed, as well as any of the notes found within the facility EMR. This means that the payer auditor will be expecting to see all notes and medications for months to years from all sources, not just the facility EMR.

If this is a charge line audit, then the payer auditor will expect to see an itemized claim in addition to this data. Because most record requests are put through the health information management department, some of these items may not be contained within the facility EMR and therefore represent a failure to receive the requested data. A data request from the payer (and Medicare/Medicaid) should always include physician notes, operative reports, nursing notes, therapy notes, ambulatory notes, pharmacy (medication administration records), physician orders, all ancillary testing results (lab, radiology, CT, MRI), progress notes from case management, and authorization information (for procedures) at a minimum. As such, many of these elements are not contained within the EMR and will have to be added to the data submitted so the payer auditor has all the information required in order to perform the analysis.

Failure to provide all the data (not just what is in the EMR) is a frequent cause of denials for which an appeal would need to be approached by the provider. One point that every facility should talk to their payer representative about is the ability to work with the auditors. This will help the facility/provider auditors become accustomed to what might be expected for documentation.

Clarity of the information

Since the creation of the EMR, it has generally been the responsibility of the facility or provider to make their own documentation templates. They are frequently assisted by information services and informatics individuals. Most of these people, while well meaning, have never audited a record. As a result, hundreds of nonessential and sometimes irrelevant data elements end up in the record. The payer auditor will receive either the .pdf or actual printed copy. In some cases, an auditor will see vital signs printed over and over again at the top of each page or laboratory results reprinted countless times; this is what an auditor refers to as "static." It is the same information that appears repeatedly throughout the record, making it hard to grasp what medically is occurring with the patient. To make this more profound, physician notes are templates that frequently do not tell the whole story that an auditor would have seen when the note was written by hand. Key elements may not be in the template, and, therefore, documentation is missing. While clinical documentation improvement teams do their best, the overall documentation may appear fragmented to the payer auditor.

Physician orders are paramount to an auditor. However, in most EMRs, the auditor may see a resident order and not an attending order. In some cases, this results in a problem, especially with an order for inpatient admission. A resident is generally not provided admitting privileges, and if the attending physician order is not cosigned soon after, it may appear tens to hundreds of pages later in the printed record and might be missed by the auditor. All attending orders should be spelled out for efficiency to ensure that the payer auditor can see everything while not getting lost in the "static."

Written plan

A written plan of care that is easy to identify in the medical record is a key requirement for all auditors, not just commercial/managed care. Additionally, current active problem lists should be present in the medical record. While HIM cannot code from a problem list, the payer auditor will use it as a benchmark against the diagnosis and procedure codes submitted for reimbursement. It cannot be used by any auditor without further verification, but it is a known method that auditors use to begin the audit process. Because of this, it fits into the "identify the standards" step of the audit process previously discussed.

With the problem list should be a written plan of care for all problems being treated. Within the plan, an auditor would expect to see the action steps to achieve the result as stated in the plan. If the steps are not reaching the stated goal of the plan, then how did the provider change the plan of care to reach an achievable goal? The plan of care will provide the medical necessity for the service. If the plan of care is missing or incomplete, then it will represent a failure of the medical record to document the necessity of the service. Additionally, auditors are trained to look for a plan of care that is poorly documented and then by some "miracle" appears only in the discharge summary. A good plan of care should speak to the severity of the problem being treated, action steps to achieve the goal stated, and an expected timeline to achieve the goal. Payers will reimburse only for medically necessary services rendered in the most appropriate status/location.

Finally, the auditor will use the problem list and look for a plan of care on all active problems. This is why it is essential to have an up-to-date problem list and not a roster of all problems that the patient has had since they were born. An accurate problem list of current ailments and goal-oriented plan of care will be your best instrument to ensure medical necessity is documented.

Surprise factors in medical records

Surprises within a medical record are very common but work to degrade the overall integrity of the document. Some examples would be a well-written emergency services note that documents the patient severity of illness states they are stable and being transferred to the floor for observation status. The next note might be from a hospitalist 20 minutes later showing the patient in acute distress, much worse than described by the emergency room physician. This could then be followed by a consultative physician stating the patient is stable during the same time period where the hospitalist states they are unstable.

Conflicting notes within relatively the same time period are "surprises." Another example of a surprise is a patient placed in observation for "respiratory symptoms" (cough, slight fever, and lowered pulse oximetry). Throughout the medical record there is no mention of sepsis. Suddenly, in the discharge summary, the physician says "sepsis," and it is coded within the sepsis code range. Clearly, this would strike an auditor as somewhat of a surprise and would make them look further.

THE FOLLOWING IS A TRUE CASE EXAMPLE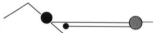

Patient admitted for upper respiratory infection:

- All laboratory tests within normal ranges
- Vital signs showed one instance of fever
- Hospitalist documents that the patient is a severe asthmatic and they are observing him to ensure he doesn't have sudden respiratory complications
- There is only one progress note from the attending physician that states, "patient stable, plan discharge tomorrow"
- The discharge summary states that the patient was admitted and treated for a course of acute respiratory failure brought on by sepsis
- The principal diagnosis was "sepsis" and "acute respiratory failure"

The auditor notes that neither acute respiratory failure nor sepsis is ever stated in the progress notes, nor is there any medical decision-making notes regarding the laboratory results. The auditor determined that this claim should be denied. The auditor also expressed concern that they had seen this before at the same facility.

The auditor took it to a superior, who ran data analytics on the facility and provider and found a significant increase in sepsis claims in the past 24 months. Accordingly, they moved the cases to the fraud audit unit, who began a thorough investigation of all sepsis and tangentially related diagnosis codes for the facility.

Surprise factors can lead to very significant audit and analytic metrics being performed by any payer. The result to the provider can be significant denials and subsequent cash disruption. Most auditors will look to see that the discharge summary contains only the same/similar information already documented within the plan of care and progress notes. Items appearing only at the time of discharge will be suspect and most likely cause a denial of the claim.

Importance of continuity and agreement

All auditors expect to see continuity in the documents they are examining. Imagine a bank auditor seeing differing amounts for the same ledger entry or a defense contractor having a test result that conflicts between multiple reporting personnel. Audit standards would not allow that in those industries, and auditors do not expect to find conflicting notes within a medical record either. With the advent of the EMR, the auditors are seeing increasing amounts of disparity compared to the older handwritten notes.

Let's take the example of physician and nursing note comparison for congruity. The physician repeatedly documents that the patient is hypoxic, cannot speak in sentences, and is limited in their activity of daily living. However, over multiple shifts and multiple nurses and therapists, we see comments such as "up walking hall with family in no apparent distress, off the floor with family to cafeteria, talking to family on the telephone in no apparent distress." Nursing vital signs show stable pulse oximetry of 94–98% over two days. This type of documentation will cause the auditor to question the validity of the record. Most likely, this will result in a request for additional data or become a denial for which the provider will require an appeal. For this reason, many payers now require case management notes for the auditor to assist with the review.

More subtle examples can be found between resident and attending documentation and between nursing shifts. These differences can occur on a singular event or multiple events but may not concern the auditor, as the plan of care is addressing how the patient is progressing and may allow the auditor to dismiss the concern in the audit but will require them to write it in an audit report as tangential finding.

Since EMR templates can create these scenarios, it is incumbent upon the internal audit staff at the facility to conduct full audits to ensure that the templates are accurately reporting and that the templates used between providers do not result in conflicts. Records should be fully printed, reviewed by a nurse reviewer, and completely vetted prior to submission to ensure that the payer receives the most accurate record for review.

Detriment of cut and paste

Cut and paste was presented as an "efficiency measure" for completing templates and bringing completeness to the notes. However, this has resulted in significant denials by all payers, government, commercial, and managed care alike. Many payers will use analytics to review the document for key words, key phrases, and similarities. This means a nurse who continually copies vital signs over by cut and paste will stand out. Physician notes that have the same phrases will be detected in the review of the scanned record. These "cut and paste" or repeat phrases will be provided to the auditor as part of the review process. Cut and paste is clearly a focus of most fraud units. The Centers for Medicare & Medicaid Services (CMS) has published a document called "Electronic Health Record" in which it states the concern with this practice (CMS, 2015).

Payers of all kinds use data analytics, natural language processing, and internal edits to look for repeating words, phrases, and numbers. When these occur, the claim will be flagged for the payer auditor for a more substantial review. If evidence is found, then the claim will likely be sent to the fraud unit for their auditors. It is incumbent upon the provider or facility to ensure that "auto fill" and "cut-and-paste" methods are not employed in the record in a way that would result in overdocumentation or overcoding or result in increased unearned reimbursement.

Put It All Together With the 5 Ws

Throughout this chapter, we have outlined what a payer auditor will require and some of the implications for not providing them what they need. The first step is to print the record to make sure all documents required to support the claim are included within the final record. Make sure any elements outside the main EMR are in fact included. Once reconciliation of all documents is performed, then the documents are to be reviewed by the auditor. The most straightforward method for a facility to ensure the payer audit group has documentation to support the claim is to pursue a method called the "5 Ws." This method was developed by Sharon Easterling, MHA, RHIA, CCS, CDIP, CRC, FAHIMA, of Recovery Analytics and models what all auditors are looking for in a record (Easterling, 2015).

According to Easterling, when CMS unveiled the 2-midnight rule and the need to certify the inpatient admission, the "5 Ws for Documentation/Auditing" were born. This laid the framework for the requirements needed to certify the admission and at the same time justify the reason for the admission (Easterling, 2015).

FIGURE 5.1 FIVE WS FOR DOCUMENTATION/AUDITING

- What are we treating? Diagnosis | Procedure (if relevant)
- Where is treatment needed? Inpatient | Outpatient (observation/surgery)
- Why is treatment needed?
    - o Why is this diagnosis acutely requiring attention?
    - o Relationship to chronicity
    - o References to requiring testing, drugs, or other interventions
    - o References in variation from baseline to current state
    - o Potential for adverse outcome
- How are we treating it?
    - o What are we actively doing requiring our level of care?
    - o Implications if not performed
- When do you think they'll get better?
    - o Expectation for stay
    - o Plan for discharge

Source: Easterling, 2015.

An auditor will expect to see a clear summary of the 5 Ws documented in the plan of care, progress note, and discharge summary. Specifically, an auditor will need to know what is being treated, in what setting, and why the patient requires treatment. The need for treatment generally can start to be found within the emergency department record. The "how" it is being treated is essential to the plan of care. What needs treated, how are we going to treat it, and when do you think the patient will get better are all key questions in a plan of care, daily progress note, consulting physician notes, therapy notes, and nursing notes to help substantiate the claim. Failure to provide any of these elements to an auditor will increase the chance of a claim denial (Easterling, 2015).

Summary

This chapter speaks to the needs of the payer auditor. Those requirements are similar to any federal payer auditor but utilize different payer guidelines. There are some cases where the guidelines match and others where they are completely divergent. Using the 5 Ws, the payer or provider auditor can quickly identify if the documentation is supportive of the guidelines, payer policies, and medical necessity. Nothing has really changed over time, just the fact that EMRs have created endless data elements, creating "static" that takes away from the documentation required by the auditor. Using the 5 Ws, every provider can ensure that despite the static produced by the EMR, the claim will be adequately supported through complete and appropriate documentation.

REFERENCES

CMS. 2015. "Electronic Health Records Provider." Retrieved from *https://www.cms.gov/Medi-care-Medicaid-Coordination/Fraud-Prevention/Medicaid-Integrity-Education/Downloads/docmat-ters-ehr-providerfactsheet.pdf.*

Easterling, S. 2015. "'The Building Blocks of Documentation' for ICD-10." Recovery Analytics, LLC. Retrieved from *http://recoveryanalyticsllc.com/the-building-blocks-of-documentation-for-icd-10/.*

Healthcare Finance. 2008. "Cigna won't pay for 'never events.'" Retrieved from *http://www.health-carefinancenews.com/news/cigna-wont-pay-never-events.*

Magellan Healthcare. 2016. "Medical Necessity Criteria Guidelines." Retrieved from *https://www.magellanprovider.com/media/1771/mnc.pdf.*

National Committee for Quality Assurance (NCQA). n.d. "HEDIS Compliance Audit Pro-gram." Retrieved from *www.ncqa.org/hedis-quality-measurement/data-reporting-services/hedis-compliance-audit-program/hedis-compliance-audit-program.*

SAS. n.d. "Big Data: What it is and why it matters." Retrieved from *www.sas.com/en_us/insights/big-data/what-is-big-data.html.*

Texas Medical Foundation (TMF), n.d. "About PEPPER." Retrieved from *https://www.pepperres-ources.org/PEPPER.*

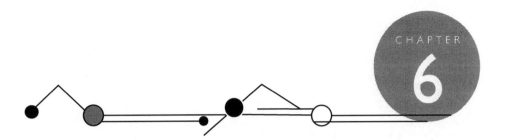

Implementing a Coding Compliance Plan

CHAPTER OBJECTIVES

- Define the steps in selecting an audit sample

- Determine the scope of the audit

- Understand what a compliance issue is

- Calculate coding accuracy

The contents of this chapter were adapted from *JustCoding's Practical Guide to Coding Management* (Dunn, 2016). Each of the prior chapters have provided the coding manager, coding auditor, and/or health information management (HIM) director with some issues that should be addressed in the coding compliance plan and schedule. One of our goals for conducting the audits is to identify opportunities that need to be mitigated before external governmental and nongovernmental reviews occur. As we see from Chapter 5's discussion, payers aggressively monitor the coding function because coding drives reimbursement. These payers capture the data on the claim, conduct trend analyses, and edit the claims for compliance with the many rules that govern coding as well as payer contractual requirements.

So, how do we, as providers and healthcare organizations, conduct our audits? We have already developed our audit schedule, which includes the topics that we have identified as having significant importance to our organization. We have hired talented staff to conduct the reviews. Now we need to do the reviews. Our first step will be to select our sample.

Selecting the Audit Sample

Sample sizes may vary depending on the purpose of the audit. A commonly recommended audit sample size is 30 cases for routine quality auditing with no known serious compliance issues. Conducting an audit of this magnitude for every coder every month can be a daunting challenge. Assess the purpose of a particular audit and consider modifying the sample size and/or allowing more time to conduct a review.

For example, when auditing for discharge disposition accuracy, review several discharges per coder every week, and then evaluate the monthly or quarterly results. Allocating enough time is a factor of the type of review being conducted. Auditing inpatient coding may take 20–40 minutes depending on the length of stay, copy-forward use, and number of conditions. It may take less time if the audit is assessing only whether the principal diagnosis was correctly assigned and that at least one comorbidity/complication (CC) or major CC (MCC) was identified. In this type of audit, the auditor is not assessing all the potential conditions that could be coded and validated (Dunn, 2016).

Spreading the review over a quarter of the year facilitates reviewing 30 cases per coder. Additionally, management should ensure that the coding performed by contracted coders is evaluated as well.

Auditors reviewing a new inexperienced coder's work may find that a sample of 30 cases is not adequate and may need to conduct a review of all cases coded until such time that the new coder demonstrates that he or she grasped the coding guidelines and is accurately assigning codes. Or, in the case of an experienced coder that is new to an organization, an audit of a substantial sample may be necessary until the auditor believes the new person understands the idiosyncrasies of the organization, its systems, and unique coding processes.

When auditing all coders for an Office of Inspector General (OIG) *Work Plan* item and nothing suggests that one or more coders have errors in the topic selected, consider reviewing a smaller sample, such as five encounters per coder. Increase the sample size to 10 for any coders with errors in the *Work Plan* issue. Continue to expand the sample if more errors are found. This auditing by exception approach limits reviews to only those coders with errors.

Samples for reporting a serious finding

Finally, depending on the purpose of the audit, the sample size may need to be increased. There is no set "statistical sample size" outlined in the self-disclosure protocol, but it does say there needs to be at least 100 items.

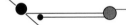

According to the OIG, when using a sample to estimate damages, the disclosing party must use a sample of at least 100 times and use the mean point estimate to calculate the damages. If a probe sample was used, those claims may be included in the 100-item sample if statistically appropriate. To avoid unreasonably large sample sizes, the self-disclosure protocol does not require a minimum precision level for the review of claims. As a result, the disclosing party may select an appropriate sample size to estimate damages as long as the sample size is at least 100 items.

Source: oig.hhs.gov/compliance/self-disclosure-info/protocol.asp.

Self-disclosure activities will come into play after an initial quality audit is conducted and it is found that a significant coding error has occurred; for example, the diagnoses were always resequenced to ensure that a diagnosis in the principal position generated the highest-weighted diagnosis-related group (DRG) regardless of whether it met the principal diagnosis definition (defined as the condition, after study, that occasioned the admission to the hospital). If such a situation occurred, the findings should be reported to the compliance officer. He or she will confer with legal counsel about how to proceed. Often, next steps will include a more extensive audit to assess the organization's exposure and to calculate the reimbursement amounts that will need to be returned to each of the DRG-paying payers. The 100-case sample would be a starting point and, for example, may be expanded to 100 cases for each payer or for each coder or for each of the most common DRGs for the organization.

Once the results are gathered, the organization may approach the regional Health and Human Services office or the payer to discuss what was found, share the anticipated overpayment, and establish a repayment approach. Often these situations may result in the OIG requiring the organization to comply with a corporate integrity agreement (CIA), which will require the organization to establish policies, procedures, and routine auditing (and reporting back to the OIG) of coding to ensure this or a similar situation does not reoccur. Providers or entities agree to the obligations, and in exchange, the OIG agrees not to seek their exclusion from participation in Medicare, Medicaid, or other federal healthcare programs. As mentioned in Chapter 1, a comprehensive CIA typically lasts five years.

A similar process would occur if the payer discovered the erroneous coding through its review of records and analysis of claim data. However, in this situation, the payer may determine which records it wishes to review and not permit you to conduct the review for them.

Selecting an unbiased sample

After determining sample size, select an unbiased sample. An unbiased sample may be selected simply by choosing cases that end in a certain digit or occur at a certain frequency. For example, the auditor may obtain a list of coder A's records for the month and audit those where the account number ends in 7. Or the auditor may choose every fifth case on the list. Either approach provides randomness in the sample.

A more sophisticated approach is the RAND function available in Excel.

One approach to using the RAND function is as follows:

Identify the account numbers that meet your audit criteria. For example, coder A coded 20 emergency department encounters this week. You now have a list of 20 account numbers (see Figure 6.1). You intend to audit five this week.

FIGURE 6.1

#	Acct. no.
1	170788
2	067877
3	891465
4	595906
5	161556
6	835387
7	114123
8	307381
9	235273
10	288857
11	219839
12	353058
13	302147
14	097092
15	805143
16	650285
17	649422
18	547794
19	962903
20	147808

FIGURE 6.2

16
11
12
15
15
1
4
18
1
20
12
5
11
8
17
7
11
13
19
4

In an Excel spreadsheet cell, type =RandBetween(1, 20). A list of whole numbers will pop up. You may need to expand the cell down the column to 20 cells to see the entire column of numbers. Twenty of the numbers are linked to the accounts listed in Figure 6.1, but these are randomly listed between 1 and 20. You will pick the first five. In this example, you will see that the first five includes a duplicated 15 (see Figure 6.2). When this occurs, you will select the first five unduplicated numbers. In this example, it would be 16, 11, 12, 15, and 1.

Go back to step one and identify those accounts that are 16, 11, 12, 15, and 1. These are the five randomly selected cases that will be reviewed for coder A.

1 = 170788

11 = 219839

12 = 353058

15 = 805143

16 = 650285

Each time you use the RAND function, it will generate a different set of random numbers for you. If you have consecutively numbered accounts, you can use the beginning and ending numbers of the range of consecutive numbers in the =RandBetween (,) formula.

Managers should select cases from the month preceding the month in which the audit is conducted. Using recent cases facilitates rebilling if an audit reveals items requiring correction.

What Should Be Audited?

We have already created our audit calendar by this point, so now we just need to assess the depth of the audit that will be conducted. Audits need to be tailored to the type of record being reviewed. Below are some factors that should be considered when determining the scope of a specific type of audit. Remember our discussion earlier about how long it may take to audit an inpatient record. If our scope is simply to assess whether the principal diagnosis was assigned correctly, the time would be less. If we assess all of the bulleted items in the DRG audit list below, the time will be more. Coding leadership and the compliance officer need to determine what is appropriate for your organization given the resources you have available.

DRG audits:

- Principal diagnosis selection and code assignment
- When two principal diagnoses are present
- Sequencing of secondary diagnoses
- Capture of all relevant conditions
- Conditions coded reflect the severity of the patient's illness, level of morbidity, and risk of mortality
- Principal procedure selection and code assignment
- Other procedure code accuracy
- Surgeon identification
- Present-on-admission accuracy
- Discharge disposition accuracy (including transfer categories)
- Facility-specific abstracting accuracy
- Presence of an order to admit to inpatient
- Challenging inpatient conditions for both coders and auditors are conditions such as encephalopathy, respiratory failure, and neoplasms
  - Auditor guidance for these conditions appears in the downloadable appendix

Ambulatory payment classifications (APC)/outpatient facility audits:

- Principal diagnosis selection and code assignment
- When two principal diagnoses are present
- Sequencing of secondary diagnoses
- Capture of all relevant conditions
- Conditions coded reflect the severity of the patient's illness, level of morbidity, and risk of mortality

- Principal procedure selection and code assignment

- Other procedure code accuracy

- Modifier usage

- Surgeon identification

For both inpatient and outpatient surgery audits, the auditor may identify postoperative complications. Distinguishing whether the condition is an expected outcome of the procedure or whether it truly is an adverse event may require additional querying on the part of the auditor and/or the coder, review by the quality or outcomes department, and possibly discussion with the organization's medical director. Some general auditor guidance is provided in the downloadable appendix.

Observation audits:

- Diagnosis accuracy

- Presence of an order to admit (and return, if applicable) to observation

- Observation hours accuracy, especially when other procedures with active monitoring occurs during the observation period

- Order to discharge from observation

- Inappropriate observation orders (such as prior to a procedure beginning)

- Factors associated with observations converted to inpatient admission, such as admission time, if the coder has responsibility for this factor

  – If the hospital is a regular inpatient prospective payment system hospital, then the "from date" on the claim in field locator 6 will have the beginning of stay as either at the time observation began or emergency department services started if prior to the observation period that was converted to an inpatient stay. For further details, see the National Uniform Billing Committee manual for the form locators.

Infusion audits:

- Similar to observation audits

- Orders for infusion and for discharge

- Infusion volumes (number of units)

- Initial and subsequent infusion admission codes
- Start and stop times noted by the nursing staff

Physician office/professional service audits:

- Evaluation/management (E/M) level assignment and modifier usage
- Capture of all relevant diagnoses, that were monitored/measured, evaluated, assessed, or treated/referred to another provider, to adequately describe the severity of the patient's illness, level of morbidity, and risk of mortality
- Procedures and modifier usage accuracy
- Cloning of notes
- Conflicts in documentation (e.g., history says patient complains of leg pain, but the musculoskeletal component of the review of systems states "musculoskeletal negative")
- Encounters consistent with supervision and "incident to" rules
- Proper usage of prolonged codes
- Capture of performance measurement (F) codes
- Assessing where the physician may be documenting conditions or procedures and determining whether these are being captured by the physician practice electronic health record for billing and problem list purposes

Hierarchical condition category (HCC) audits:

- Documentation appropriately authenticated
- Documentation legible
- Diagnosis coding accuracy and specificity
- Diagnoses coded are from face-to-face provider encounters

Other audits:

- Reviewing UB-04s for any CPT®/HCPCS that may be hardcoded in the 1xxxx to 6xxxx and 9xxxx series to ensure that the procedure codes are correct and to evaluate whether these should be soft-coded.

Audit Timing

As discussed earlier, the time to conduct an audit will vary based on the scope. Based on our experience, to conduct a comprehensive scope, the audit time is slightly more than the time to do the coding, because the auditor must ascertain where the coder found a diagnosis, procedure, or specific component of the diagnosis or procedure code that the auditor did not see when the auditor reviewed the record. Plus, you need to factor in the additional time to record the findings and prepare a summary report.

FIGURE 6.3 AUDIT TIMES

At the 2017 AHIMA Convention, the following audit times were reported by Banner Health's Senior Coding Director, Jannifer Owens.

Audit type	Minutes/each	Audit type	Minutes/each
Inpatient	18	Claims review	7
Emergency department	7	Insurance denials	10
CDI mismatch	10	State data	6

Source: Owens, Jannifer. Productivity Standards for Auditors in ICD-10. AHIMA National Convention. 10/2017.

Experience reported from the First Class Solutions, Inc., audit team for some recent audits appears below:

Record type	Time	Comments
Inpatient	58.4 min.; 2.4 min. per code.	Tertiary, teaching, facility; EHR; audit, share changes, enter data; does not include time for summary session or final report preparation.
Observation and interventional radiology	25 min.; 2.5 min. per code	Tertiary, teaching, facility; EHR; does not include time for summary session or final report preparation.
Professional E/M (ED)	9.4 min.	Scanned encounters; includes final report preparation; no summary session time.

FIGURE 6.3 AUDIT TIMES (CONT.)

Record type	Time	Comments
Professional E/M, diagnosis, CPT (office)	10.1 min.	EHR; does not include time for summary session or final report preparation.
Professional CPT (operative reports)	9.2 min.	Scanned documents; includes report; excludes summary session.

Source: Rose T. Dunn. Reprinted with permission.

Environmental conditions will impact the time it takes to perform the audits. Similar to the coding environment, the auditing environment must be quiet, with little or no distractions, comfortable temperature-wise, with access to reference materials, ergonomically designed furniture, and at minimum a dual-monitor computer system setup. Some auditors actually prefer quad-monitors to allow them to have the record up on two screens, the encoder on a third screen, and their audit form on the fourth. Others continue to use paper forms for their audit form purposes and then enter their findings into their audit report from the forms. An example of an audit report spreadsheet appears in Figure 6.4 and comparative report in Figure 6.5.

FIGURE 6.4 SAMPLE AUDIT SPREADSHEET

Acct. No.	Original Dx Codes	Revised Dx Codes	% Same	Original Proc Codes	Revised Proc Codes	% Same	Original DRG	Revised DRG	Value Change	Original APCs	Revised APCs	Value Change

Coder:

Coding Accuracy:

Financial Value Change:

Finding Summary an Recommendations: (In this area, the auditor would summarize the findings. Categorizing issues identified, such as sequencing errors, coding guidelines error, insufficient documentation to support code, biopsy vs. excision, unbundled codes, etc. with an explanation of the correct coding practice.)

Other Comments:

Source: Rose T. Dunn. Reprinted with permission.

FIGURE 6.5 COMPARATIVE SUMMARY

Coder	Coding Accuracy	DRG Value Change	APC Value Change	Education Opportunities
Coder 1				
Coder 2				
Coder 3				
Coder 4				

Source: Rose T. Dunn. Reprinted with permission.

Identifying Compliance-Related Issues

For all audits, observation of any compliance-related issues should be noted and reported as appropriate. When considering compliance issues, think like an external auditor (see Chapter 5). What would raise a question in an external auditor's mind? These issues may include:

- Untimely documentation, that is, documentation that arrived in the record after the case was coded. This situation may also signal inappropriate charges if a test was performed and then results were reported after the patient was discharged. The concern would be whether the test was necessary if the patient was treated and discharged without the results.

- Questionable documentation: Documentation that may be questionable includes repeated copy-forward documentation with no changes or when multiple encounters are created on the same date, especially when that date is after all of the encounters, such as a supervising physician's statement stating she or he was present and examined the patient, but the entry was created after discharge for each of the encounters documented by a resident.

- Injuries or infections that do not appear in the physician's notes or discharge summary but are addressed in nursing notes or other documentation or reports.

The Essential Guide to Coding Audits

- Biting: Biting is a term used to describe when one provider criticizes another provider's care, treatment plan, or approach, openly in the patient's record. The criticizer "bites" the other person (Dunn, 2016).

Calculating Coding Accuracy

No coding expectation would be complete without a quality standard. Quality coding consists of assigning:

- The correct code or codes to denote the condition or procedure
- The correct number of codes to describe the encounter accurately
- For inpatients, the appropriate present-on-admission (POA) indicator for the conditions coded and discharge disposition
- For surgical episodes, the surgery date and surgeon
- Any additional elements that coding management deems appropriate (i.e., presence of admit to inpatient or observation order, reason for the visit, etc.)

Ideally, coders would assign codes accurately 100% of the time. However, challenges such as inadequate or incomplete physician documentation, illegibility of paper documents, conflicting coding rules, and human error make this standard difficult to achieve. This is why a coding accuracy expectation of 95% is reasonable to consider.

Next, we must calculate the accuracy rate.

Code-over-code: In the code-over-code calculation, include any coding error, such as revised, added, or deleted codes. A revised code could include the modification of a digit or character or a modifier. The formula for this accuracy calculation is to:

Divide the total number of accurate codes assigned originally by the coder by the total accurate codes as determined by the reviewer.

Example: The coder assigned 37 codes for the 10 discharges reviewed by the reviewer (auditor). The coder coded two symptoms that were included in other coder, failed to select the most specific code for one of the diagnosis codes, missed assigning codes for two chronic conditions that were treated during the stays, and failed to add required digits to two diagnoses. The coder assigned 32 codes correctly. However, the reviewer found two missed codes. So, the accuracy rate is based on 39 possible correct codes and is 32/39 or 82%.

However, there are times when a coder may code excess codes, such as symptoms that are considered implied in the specific diagnosis, or more incorrect codes than the total auditor codes. When this happens, the accuracy rate needs to reflect the overall coder's accuracy. In this scenario, excess incorrect coders must be subtracted from the coder's correct codes.

Example: Coder reported eight codes, and two were incorrect. Auditor coded six codes. If we use the formula above, it would be: 6/6 or 100%.

However, the coder had two incorrect codes. So, the results need to be adjusted for the coder's errors: (6 − 2)/6, or 67% code-over-code accuracy.

Some auditors prefer to report the results based on auditor findings rather than a coder's incorrect codes. So, for the above scenario, the formula would be: 6/(6 + 2) or 75%.

You can see how this formula may not precisely describe the coder's accuracy.

Organizations must determine how it will handle those excess codes that are symptoms. Symptoms may not necessarily be appropriate to code but may be necessary to support medical necessity of a test or procedure that was performed during the episode of care or encounter.

Regardless of the formula that you choose, it is important to use your code-over-code accuracy calculation consistently to be able to demonstrate trends in coder performance over time.

Case-over-case: Case-over-case calculation or, as some call it, reimbursement accuracy, involves determining whether coding changes would have resulted in a DRG or APC change. This approach is often used to determine reimbursement accuracy. The formula for this accuracy calculation is to:

> *Divide the total cases in which the coder-assigned codes resulted in the correct DRG (or APC) by the total number of cases reviewed.*

Example: Assume that 30 inpatient cases were reviewed and that the correct DRG was determined for 27 of them. The DRG accuracy rate based on the case-over-case approach is 27/30 or 90%.

This approach also is used for APCs and E/M accuracy calculations.

Example: Assume that 30 emergency department cases were reviewed for facility coding accuracy and APC capture. According to the reviewer's case review, the 30 outpatient cases qualified for 46 APCs. Based on the quality review, the coder's coding generated only 43 APCs. APC accuracy: 43/46 or 93%.

Assume the E/M level for a sample of 30 encounters was correctly chosen for 27 of them. 27/30 = 90% accuracy.

Some organizations take this approach one step further by defining accuracy of principal diagnosis and procedure assignment. For example, consider a review of 30 discharges representing 15 medical discharges with no procedures and 15 surgical discharges. The principal diagnosis was coded and sequenced accurately in 28 discharges, and the principal procedure was accurately coded and sequenced in all cases. This example includes 30 possible correct principal diagnoses and 15 possible correct principal procedures. The accuracy rate for "principal" code assignment in this example is (28 + 15)/45 or 96%. Additionally, this is the accuracy rate for sequencing as well. Further refinement of this calculation reveals an accuracy rate of 28/30 or 93% for principal diagnoses and 100% (15/15) for principal procedures.

This approach can be used for POA accuracy and discharge disposition accuracy as well.

How the two methods compare

The code-over-code approach helps identify weaknesses specific to individual coders, but it is a more complex calculation. Compliance departments tend to prefer this accuracy calculation, as does the coder since it gives the coder credit for the codes correctly assigned.

The case-over-case formula is easier to calculate and speaks to the reimbursement risk associated with the coding team, specifically when used for DRG and APC accuracy. If the principal diagnosis is not assigned correctly, the likelihood of DRG accuracy is lower. However, for outpatients, both methods could signal reimbursement risk because CPT codes drive APCs and diagnosis codes drive HCCs. If a code is missing, reimbursement may be affected.

Each organization should establish accuracy expectations and the method it will use to measure accuracy. The accuracy rate should be based on what is expected rather than the current staff's competency. Don't establish a low accuracy rate because the team is learning to code.

Consider how coding accuracy affects reimbursement for the emergency department encounters. Assume an organization bills 10,000 encounters annually. A coding quality audit reveals an APC accuracy rate of 94%. This accuracy rate translates to a loss of revenue averaging $150 per encounter for the 100 sample cases. Multiplying the total number of emergency department cases by the average loss (10,000 x $150) projects an annual loss of $1.5 million.

Quality reviews should not stop at codes assigned. Coders are often responsible for abstracting data from patient records and entering them along with the codes into the abstracting system. The abstracting system feeds the claims system and populates databases for quality improvement, decision support, and credentialing applications. If the coding is perfect but the abstracting contains transpositions or other errors, the reimbursement expected will not be achieved. The quality of the abstracted data elements, which may include dates of surgeries and consultations, the type of anesthesia, presence of an unexpected occurrence, blood types, Apgar score, POA indicators, and discharge disposition, should undergo periodic assessment.

Facilitating coding integrity is a responsibility of the coding manager. Developing a plan and implementing a program to improve the quality of coding will support the data needs of multiple departments within your organization as well as contribute to your organization achieving its entitled reimbursement. At the same time, providing appropriate resources and education and feedback to the coding team will develop a workforce committed to the quality goal.

Providing Audit Feedback

Providing feedback to the coders or practitioners audited is one of the most important steps of the auditing process. As discussed earlier, this is not a "gotcha" conversation. The feedback should be educational in its approach and ideally the auditor will have the cases available to show the coder or practitioner how the auditor arrived at his or her determination. This allows the coder or practitioner to review the case and show what documentation they used to apply their codes.

The auditor should be prepared to identify where documentation may not have been present when the coder coded the case. Additionally, having ready access to the *Official Guidelines for Coding and Reporting*, the 1995 and 1997 E/M coding guidelines, and any facility-specific guidelines can help explain why the auditor's code selection is aligned more closely with the rules than the codes selected by the coder or practitioner.

However, since coding is not always black and white, auditors need to be ready to compromise when the coder or practitioner's rationale is appropriate.

We delve deeper into providing feedback to providers and coders in Chapter 8.

Sharing the findings with others

In addition to the coders and practitioners audited, the coding compliance auditor may be required to present and submit a summary to leadership at the compliance committee. When doing so, the auditor should avoid the use of codes and coding jargon, as the leaders will lose interest if they do not understand the terms or have coding skills. Your summary should include the following points:

- What was the objective of the audit? Was the audit initiated to address a high-risk or known problem, routine compliance, regulatory compliance, financial, etc.?

- How many cases were reviewed and what percentage does the sample represent of the month, quarter, year, etc.? Be able to verbally explain how you chose the sample, if asked.

- Avoid subjective comments, and state only the objective facts. Statements such as "I feel" or "It was assumed" should be avoided. The coding report is a report of the coding accuracy findings. It is not a vehicle for "throwing another department under the bus." For example, if 100 cases were requested from the information systems report writer and the report writer provided only 75 cases when there were actually enough cases in the universe to provide you with 100, the statement in the report would be simply "100 cases were requested for this review; 75 cases were provided." If the compliance department asks why, then you can respond.

- What were the findings? Findings should be stated positively; for example, instead of stating that there was an 8% error rate, state that there was a 92% accuracy rate. It's OK to state that the goal is 95%.
- Use bullet points rather than paragraphs for ease of reading.
- Identify the top two or three issues and recommendations from the review.
- Use graphs or charts to provide variety in the content of your report and facilitate understanding the findings for those individuals who prefer visuals rather than text.
- Close with the next planned steps.

Closing the Audit Process

The final step of the process is to correct the data that was submitted to payers. It is recommended that organizations rebill accounts found to have coding errors regardless of whether discovery of the error results in additional payment or a reduced payment. The reason for rebilling an account with a coding error that does not result in a change of payment is to ensure that the patient's file with the insurer accurately reflects the conditions for which they were treated.

At minimum, cases where the organization was overpaid for a service due to identified coding or charging errors should be rebilled and a refund made of the original payment. As discussed in Chapter 4, the refunding of overpayments should occur within 60 days of finding the error. See the February 11, 2016, CMS notice "Medicare Reporting and Returning of Self-Identified Overpayments" available on CMS' website at *www.cms.gov/Newsroom/MediaRelease-Database/Fact-sheets/2016-Fact-sheets-items/2016-02-11.html*.

Often when accounts are rebilled, the payer may require a copy of the record to accompany the rebilled to them. In collaboration with the compliance officer and patient financial services, create a cover letter that will accompany any record copies for rebilled accounts. It is recommended that the letter indicate the refund is being provided as a result of the organization's routine compliance reviews. If legal counsel is involved, your attorney will draft a letter to accompany the refund.

Summary

Conducting an audit for every coder, including your contracted coders, every month can be a daunting challenge. Assess the purpose of a particular audit and consider spreading the audit over several weeks or modifying the sample size and/or allowing more time to conduct a review. The time to conduct an audit will vary based on the scope.

After determining the sample size, select an unbiased sample. An unbiased sample may be chosen in several ways. For all audits, observation of any compliance-related issues should be noted and reported. However, the goal of auditing should be to compare your coding accuracy against your stated expectation. The results of the audit should be assessed against their effects on your organization's reimbursement.

Providing feedback to the coders or practitioners audited is one of the most important steps of the auditing process, because they will be interested in how well they are meeting the organization's expectations and what they need to do to improve. However, since coding is not always black or white, auditors need to be ready to compromise when the coder or practitioner's rationale is appropriate.

The final step of the process is to correct the data that was submitted to payers, which may include refunding payments and rebilling accounts.

REFERENCE

Dunn, R.T. 2016. *JustCoding's Practical Guide to Coding Management*. Middleton, MA: HCPro, Inc.

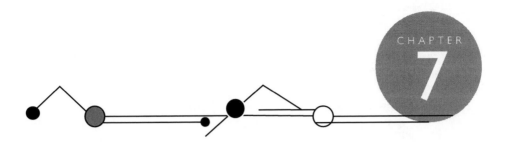

The Coding Auditor's Role in Denial Management

CHAPTER OBJECTIVES

- Developing a denial management process

- Tracking and addressing common denials

- Preparing a valid coding appeal of a coding denial

- Understanding how electronic health records (EHR) may increase exposure to denials

- Helping physicians achieve accurate Evaluation and Management levels

Although many organizations have implemented processes to ensure revenue and data integrity in their daily claims creation and submission activities, some claim denials will continue to occur. Some of these denials may be for a single item on the claim or even the entire claim. Denials can be challenging, and some may be considered unpreventable. It is these denials that continue to incent those driving the denial management process to find a way to prevent them.

The Denial Management Process

Many organizations have a denial management process. It may be informal or formal with an appointed committee.

A formal committee will often include representatives such as:

- Patient financial services
- Health information management/coding
- Scheduling
- Registration
- Utilization and/or case management and discharge planning
- Compliance/legal counsel
- Departments contributing charges to the claim
- Departments representing source of denials
- Information technology and decision support
- Practice management
- Six Sigma black belt holder
- Chief financial officer

Regardless of the structure, coding should participate in the denial management process.

Common Denial Errors

Each organization needs to assess the reasons, frequency, and sources of their denials. Most are human-related and therefore can be addressed through education and management oversight. Common reasons for denials are listed below. Some are due to the coding function and therefore serve as issues that could be monitored by the auditing function.

Submitted to the wrong payer or at the wrong address

This cause or source of this type of denial is usually the front-end staff, such as preadmission, scheduling, and access personnel.

Coordination of benefits

Coordination of benefits (COB) is a complex formula that defines which payer will be primary, that is, principal, for paying the major portion of the claimed expenses. CMS defines COB as allowing plans that provide health and/or prescription coverage for a person with Medicare to determine their respective payment responsibilities. For example, the insured can determine which insurance plan has the primary payment responsibility and the extent to which the other plans will contribute when an individual is covered by more than one plan (CMS, 2016).

The source of denials related to COB, similarly, may be related to the accurate capture of payer information by the front-end staff as well as ensuring systems, including that an organization's clearinghouses are properly designed to identify the primary payer (CMS, 2016).

Ineligibility/noncovered benefits/noncoverage

Validating a patient's coverage and eligibility to receive services is principally the function of the preadmission and scheduling processes.

Duplicate claim

This denial is the presence of more than one claim for the same service on the same date of service being submitted to the payer. This denial is due to the lack of back-end system editing.

Missing or incorrect information

A denial for missing or incorrect information may be sourced in many revenue cycle functions, including coding. Missing elements that could result from coding are the surgeon's name or surgery date, and incorrect information may be an incorrect health insurance identification number.

Medical necessity

As we have discussed, the need to understand the medical necessity coverage determinations (local and national) and understanding how to code documented conditions to support medical necessity is a coding duty. However, ensuring that advance beneficiary notices are obtained before a service that is supported by the documented conditions is a front-end obligation. We will discuss this further in this chapter and how coding can assist.

Technical

Technical denials are often preventable. According to the insurer Humana, a technical denial is a denial of the entire paid amount of a claim in instances when the care provided to a member cannot be substantiated due to a healthcare provider's nonresponse to Humana's requests for medical records, itemized bills, documents, etc. (Humana, n.d.).

Medicare calls these denials additional development requests (ADR). When a claim is selected for medical review, a medical review ADR is generated requesting medical documentation be submitted to ensure payment is appropriate. Documentation must be received by the payer within a certain time period for review and payment determination. Healthcare staff often call these ADRs. While coding is not directly responsible for this denial, the coding and audit functions can help avoid denials by identifying occurrences of lack of documented evidence of charges appearing on the claim.

Carveouts

This denial is for a portion or line of the claim. Examples include denying a day of service that is not considered necessary because the organization does not perform testing on Sunday and the patient was required to spend an additional night in the hospital. Another denial could occur when certain services are covered under another payer arrangement.

Coding (including revenue and chargemaster description codes)

This is a broad category of denials and relates to any codes on the claim, including diagnosis, procedure, revenue, discharge disposition, and present-on-admission codes.

Denials will be triggered by payers (commercial and governmental). Payers have an obligation to ensure the clinical documentation supports the services for which they are paying. They look for unusual patterns and practices that are not compliant with the payer's medical and coverage policies.

Coding and Denials

When denials are due to coding or codes, such as those from the chargemaster, it is necessary for coding leadership to provide input, prepare appeals, and track coding-related denials. Denials may identify chargemaster description voids and errors. Coding leadership can assist the chargemaster team with updates and proper assignment of CPT-4® codes. Coding audits may identify incorrect or duplicate CDM codes appearing on the claim. These may be due to inappropriate hard coding as discussed in Chapter 2, or it may be a system setting.

For example, the operating room (OR) scheduling system may capture a CPT code to prompt the OR staff to assign an adequate amount of OR time, gather the appropriate supplies, and allocate staff. However, if the scheduling system automatically populates the code section of the UB-04 or CMS 1500 (claim forms), the code may not be complete (lacking modifiers) or, more seriously, be inaccurate. The coding compliance auditor is in a position to identify these issues when conducting reviews. All coding auditor reviews should compare the codes assigned by the coding staff to the claim and, at the same time, review any other ICD-10 and CPT codes appearing on the claim.

Coding denials may be due to several reasons, but one item the coding auditor should consider is whether the coding could have been more precise if a query was issued or responded to by a physician. Query opportunities may be available during the encounter by individuals performing concurrent coding, clinical documentation improvement (CDI), and case management. When the coding compliance auditor identifies documentation that lacks precision or does not reflect conditions that clinically are being addressed, there is an opportunity to collaborate with other departments to contribute to clinical data integrity. This is not a reason to completely delegate the responsibility of physician queries to the coding professional, but it is an opportunity to enhance the collaborating department's performance. We could assume that concurrent coding is staffed by coding professionals reporting to the same leadership as the coders assigning the final codes after discharge. The responsibility of CDI specialists is to secure documentation precision and completeness.

However, the role of case management is to ensure the services and stay are covered and that the patient has the support services necessary and the appropriate level of care to address the patient's conditions. There is nothing in that role that speaks to "coding." The case manager may use codes to support a requested length of stay, and the case manager will need clinical documentation to support his or her discussion with payers and service providers. Identifying a few documentation items that will help the case manager and the coder, such as conditions being treated clinically but not documented or conditions that qualify for inpatient or outpatient status, will equally benefit the case manager and the coding team.

Appealing Denials

After review of the payer's denial reason and medical record, the coding compliance auditor should prepare the appeal if he or she remains in agreement with the codes submitted.

Preparing appeals requires providing sufficient information to sway the opinion of the payer auditors. When submitting the proof, highlight information that may have been overlooked or considered by the payer's initial reviewer. One characteristic of a good appeal process includes timeliness. Waiting until the last day to submit an appeal may result in leaving out key facts that provide the important proof that the organization is entitled to the payment.

As recommended earlier, ensuring that the complete record is provided and tagging the pages that provide the source of the information on which codes were based are important steps. The appeal should be based on a payer's misinterpretation, not your error. Always research the background of the denial before appealing so that the information submitted is pertinent to the denial reason. Include reference materials such as direct quotes from *Coding Clinic* or the *Official Guidelines for Coding and Reporting*. If the denial is from a nongovernmental payer, include references from the payer's advisory newsletters, if available.

Tracking to Enhance Performance

The coding compliance auditor should also track the reason for coding-related denials, including the:

- Diagnosis
- Procedure
- Evaluation/management (E/M) level
- Coder
- Physician
- Dollar amount
- Payer

Each of these items may lead to seeing a trend. Diagnosis denials may be triggered from multiple principal diagnoses present at the time of admission, but one results in a higher reimbursement than the other. Procedure denials may be the result of different procedure codes being submitted by the surgeon and the facility. This may signal a need to collaborate with certain proceduralists and surgeons about the proper code to submit. Tracking E/M level denials along with the provider may identify an education opportunity for the provider as well as the use of autofilling templates in the EHR that result in hiking an E/M level, sometimes unbeknownst to the provider. Monitoring the frequency of denials by the coder and by the physician may also provide education opportunities. The time spent to capture the data will have a value over time and can demonstrate a reduction in denials or denied dollars resulting from codes.

Second Look and Comparisons

Coding compliance auditors may be responsible for conducting "second looks." Second looks are reviews of inpatient cases coded by the coding team that lack a comorbidity/complication (CC) or major CC (MCC). During this second review, the auditor is not only attempting to find an uncoded CC or MCC but is also assessing whether the coder's coding is accurate, sequenced appropriately, and eligible for a physician query and that there are no unsupported charges or duplicate codes on the claim. Doing so provides additional assurances that a payer will not find a reason to deny the case for a clinical coding-related issue.

As may be apparent from other comments in this book, the auditor's role is broader than assessing coding by the coding team and involves capturing data to identify trends that may require further investigation before your payers or the external auditors, such as the Recovery Audit Contractors, see the trends. For example, it may be beneficial to monitor coding opportunities that may exist with Medicare-severity diagnosis-related group (MS-DRG) pairs and triplets. This would be a natural partner of second-look reviews. Monitoring the frequency when a DRG is converted from one without a CC or MCC to one with a CC or an MCC has a direct impact on the case-mix index and reimbursement.

The monitoring effort could also identify opportunities for CDI and case management collaboration. Directions for comparing the organization's distribution of DRGs within a pair or triplet to the MedPAR data is available through *CMS.gov* and by using Tables 7A and 7B on the website.

According to "Data Analysis Trending to Identify MS-DRG Pair/Triplet Documentation and Coding Opportunities," instructions are:

1. Add the total number of discharges per MS-DRG in the twin or triplet of the CMS table

2. Divide each MS-DRG into the twin/triplet total

3. Equals the percent to total per MS-DRG discharge

4. Use the same formula using your facility data (Drake, Land, Poleon, 2017)

Using the comparison table, determine where there may be opportunities to:

- Provide essential education for the coding and CDI teams
- Mine the facility data by coder and create individual frequency data by MS-DRG to identify variations between coders
- Promote collaborative efforts between coding, CDI, and case management to improve and legitimately exceed the average nationwide

If the latter is pursued, the coding auditor, CDI, and case management teams should report their plans and efforts at the performance improvement and compliance committees. Be aware that if your performance excessively exceeds the norm, then payers may more closely monitor your claims. Norms are available for E/M codes as well on the CMS website at *https://www.cms.gov/apps/ama/license.asp?file=/Research-Statistics-Data-and-Systems/Statistics-Trends-and-Reports/MedicareFeeforSvcPartsAB/Downloads/EMSpecialty2016.pdf.*

The data from this site are displayed by E/M code and specialty. See Figure 7.1. When the compliance auditor is conducting reviews of a physician, the norms, otherwise known as the E/M bell curve for the specialty, should be compiled. An example of an E/M curve for a general surgery appears in Figure 7.2. Capture the actual experience of each of your providers and compare side by side.

When investigating audit opportunities, these bell curve comparisons may identify skewing of the curve to the right or left or a much higher frequency of one or more levels than the national curve. Our goal should be to find outliers before our payers find them in their claims analytics software and request to conduct their own audit of our providers. Obtain from the practice management system an Excel data dump of E/M level codes, account numbers, dates of service, and provider names. This will allow the data to be sorted by provider and E/M level and will calculate the volumes of each E/M level for the provider and graph the provider's bell curve. This allows the auditor to reveal whether there is a variation from national averages. The additional advantage is that the spreadsheet now provides encounters within the E/M levels that appear to be at variance to be audited to determine whether there is inappropriate coding, insufficient documentation, education necessary, and rebilling required.

FIGURE 7.1 EXCERPT OF MEDICARE PART B PHYSICIAN/SUPPLIER NATIONAL DATA

MEDICARE PART B PHYSICIAN/SUPPLIER NATIONAL DATA CY2016
EVALUATION AND MANAGEMENT CODES BY SPECIALTY
Codes Copyrighted By American Medical Association

Data have been screened to meet CMS privacy guidelines
Sum of columns may not equal total

HCPCS CODE	SPECIALTY	ALLOWED SERVICES	ALLOWED CHARGES	PAYMENT AMOUNT
	General Practice	1,237	51,685	34,409
	General Surgery	23,455	922,067	636,921
	Allergy/Immunology	263	9,784	7,174
	Otolaryngology	7,524	307,250	202,230
	Anesthesiology	2,900	88,152	65,697
	Cardiology	2,242	88,585	62,416
	Dermatology	76,864	3,235,204	2,061,712
	Family Practice	10,086	410,540	241,212
	Interventional Pain Management	238	9,642	6,918
	Gastroenterology	6,089	247,857	162,640
	Internal Medicine	6,125	250,377	156,146
	Osteopathic Manipulative Medicine	101	4,354	2,867
	Neurology	2,567	101,886	72,676
	Neurosurgery	4,535	166,253	120,616
	Obstetrics/Gynecology	5,863	233,804	157,954
	Hospice and Palliative Care	39	1,353	984
	Ophthalmology	2,659	108,329	68,792
	Oral Surgery (dentists only)	4,505	184,639	126,652
	Orthopedic Surgery	11,939	475,164	325,374
	Cardiac Electrophysiology	358	14,767	9,876
	Pathology	2,512	103,925	79,540
	Sports Medicine	183	6,735	4,711
99201	Plastic and Reconstructive Surgery	8,724	342,870	235,101
	Physical Medicine and Rehabilitation	3,168	127,815	92,959
	Psychiatry	660	22,380	14,382
	Colorectal Surgery (formerly proctology)	1,673	68,781	44,569
	Pulmonary Disease	737	26,995	18,878
	Diagnostic Radiology	2,255	80,648	59,677
	Thoracic Surgery	1,332	50,301	37,382
	Urology	5,292	207,835	143,433
	Nuclear Medicine	266	11,716	8,879
	Pediatric Medicine	296	10,934	7,585
	Geriatric Medicine	108	4,255	2,796
	Nephrology	416	16,268	11,547
	Hand Surgery	1,193	49,045	32,801
	Optometry	3,298	134,180	83,614
	Certified Nurse Midwife (effective July 1, 1988)	149	5,821	3,864
	Certified Registered Nurse Anesthetist (CRNA)	53	1,468	1,072
	Infectious Disease	416	15,771	11,033
	Endocrinology	338	14,251	10,188
	Podiatry	15,366	639,683	428,752
	Nurse Practitioner	21,287	737,327	467,902
	Rheumatology	448	18,213	11,944
	Clinical Laboratory (Billing Independently)	573	25,123	18,600

FIGURE 7.2 EXAMPLE OF A BELL CURVE FOR A GENERAL SURGERY'S NATIONAL DATA

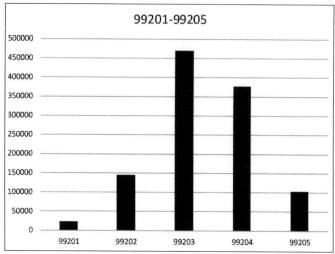

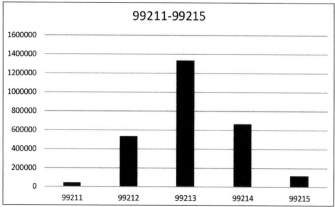

General Surgery CMS Data CY 2016 Office Visits	
99201	23455
99202	145296
99203	470777
99204	377180
99205	103894
99211	41734
99212	530130
99213	666964
99214	666964
99215	119438

Source: CMS

EHR Impact on Provider Denials

In an effort to help physicians with their documentation, the electronic health record (EHR) can be set up to prompt the provider to capture certain documentation. Occasionally, the setup includes autofilling fields assuming that the provider has assessed certain systems or conditions and permits copy-forward of prior documentation. Unfortunately, the autopopulation features of EHRs often incorporate canned documentation that may be more detailed than what had actually been discussed between the patient and provider.

Payers review the diagnoses and compare to the examination performed. If an excessive exam is performed for a simple condition, it may raise the E/M level superficially. The higher E/M level will be considered unjustified and denied. CMS, Comprehensive Error Rate Testing, Recovery Audit Contractors, Office of Inspector General, and commercial payers perceive risk with E/M leveling and EHRs, so profiling of providers against others in the same specialty is conducted to identify variations.

Reasons for physician denials are similar to those we discussed earlier but also include:

- Incorrectly coding a visit as a new patient when the patient is considered established. In order for a patient to be considered a new patient, the patient may not have received any professional services within the past three years from any provider of the same specialty within the practice and must meet the E/M elements of history, exam, and medical decision-making.
- Visit level does not meet medical necessity as discussed above.
- Inadequate support for a consultation. Consultations require specific documentation. There must be a physician request for an opinion or advice, the request must state a reason to justify the need for a consultation, the consultant must

render an assessment of the patient and create a written report of their findings and recommendation—otherwise known as the Four Rs.

- Lack of sufficient documentation to support time-based encounters.
- Maintenance therapy by chiropractors.

Keeping a pulse on trends in physician/provider denials allows the coding compliance auditor to proactively review cases to identify vulnerabilities existing within the physician practice. If these denials are occurring within the practice, then reactive auditing may be necessary to reduce denial occurrences for the practice.

The coding compliance auditor's role is to periodically review the E/M levels being claimed for the organization's employed providers. When conducting these reviews, the auditor should assess whether all documented diagnoses have been coded and submitted on the claim. Doing so helps to demonstrate the complexity of the care process for the individual patient. Procedure codes should be assessed as well to ensure that current procedure codes are being used. Additionally, with the increased attention being given to transparency and public profiles by insurers and patients, there is an opportunity for the coding auditor to teach coders how to provide clinical documentation guidance to providers that may more accurately depict the complexity of an outpatient's condition.

When scenarios surface like the ones described above, the auditor may need to work with information technology and the provider to reset the parameters of the EHR in order to avoid overbilling the service level and exposing the organization to external payer audits and denials. We should be educating providers to ensure the services rendered are based on the medical necessity of the visit and that services are properly documented and categorized as new, established, or consult. Ideally, the physician's notes should tell the story about the patient's condition and how it will be addressed.

Summary

The coding compliance auditor plays an important role in denial management. Identifying trends and addressing those through ongoing monitoring, second reviews, charge and documentation comparisons, system modifications, and education of staff involved is necessary to combat continued denials. Occasionally, denials are not justified. When this occurs, auditors should participate in the preparation of appeals using the content of the medical record and official reference materials that justify the coding that was submitted.

REFERENCES

CMS. 2016. "Coordination of Benefits." CMS. Retrieved from *https://www.cms.gov/Medicare/ Coordination-of-Benefits-and-Recovery/Coordination-of-Benefits-and-Recovery-Overview/Coordina- tion-of-Benefits/Coordination-of-Benefits.html.*

Drake, S., Land, D., Poleon, C. 2017. "Data Analysis Trending to Identify MS-DRG Pair/Triplet Docu- mentation and Coding Opportunities." AHIMA 2017 National Convention.

Humana. n.d. "Humana Provider Payment Integrity Technical Denial Policy." Retrieved from *https://www.humana.com/provider/support/claims/financial-recovery/technical-denial.*

CHAPTER 8

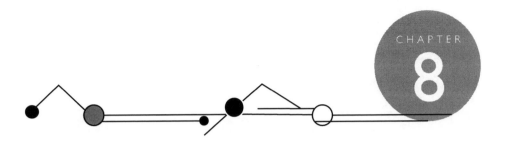

Communicating Results to Providers and Coders

CHAPTER OBJECTIVES

- Identify the auditor expectations when providing feedback to coders and providers
- Discuss approaches for presenting the findings
- Explain why text and visuals are important for reader comprehension
- Recognize that the auditor can and should go beyond the auditing role

In Chapter 6, we talked about presenting findings to providers and coders. Having a face-to-face meeting with the individual allows you to gauge body language and comprehension of the information you are conveying. The primary purpose of this discussion is to provide feedback that is educational in format and will trigger behavior change that will improve documentation specificity and/or coding accuracy.

The tone of the discussion should convey compassion for the coder and physician's feelings about having their work reviewed by another. When I conduct assessments, I always try to put myself in the shoes of those being reviewed and often try to lighten up the environment with a statement like, "I know how you may be feeling; it's like when my mother-in-law comes to my house and rearranges my husband's underwear drawer!"

For purposes of this chapter, I asked some of the First Class Solutions, Inc.'s coding audit team members about their approaches with staff.

Here is what they said:

> *I find it really difficult to explain the details in writing. In think in addition to the report, it is best to meet with the provider [face to face]. Even when I reference a CMS tool in the report, I don't think that it fully explains the specific issues [I am seeing] in their documentation, e.g., the differences between a 99212 and 99213/medical decision-making. Having the discussion in person is really useful.* —Ben Burton, JD, RHIA, CPC, CRC, CHPS, CHC, HIM consultant

> *I think it is important to approach clinicians with audit results under the auspice of 'feedback.' A benefit to such is that it seems more collegial to providers and encourages them to engage in dialogue and provide their thoughts and rational and, at times, additional information. We often find that providers have general misconceptions about documentation and coding and will share 'I've always been told....' As auditors/educators, we can then discuss common misconceptions and utilize tools and resources to demonstrate and support points or recommendations. Providers often respond well to literature or guidance from their professional association and societies, so when appropriate, I check for such resources and share them with the provider.* —Sally Frese, MSN, RN, CPC, ProFee compliance consultant

> *Meeting with the providers face to face to discuss the results is best. We can actually walk through encounters with them, have them code*

their own notes while we're there, and also see how they document within their EHR. Sometimes one keystroke is the cause of an upcode or downcode situation. As we all know, however, it is difficult scheduling time with providers, so, if face to face is not an option, do a conference call or GoToMeeting call so you can 'talk' and 'show' them the findings. —David Vence, MHI, MA, RHIA, CPC, assistant vice president, ProFee compliance consultant

For E/M audits where the physician does his own coding, it is always a good idea to sit with the physician, if possible, to go over some of the notes with them and show them where they could have documented more or even worded it a little differently. The physicians seem to enjoy this approach (as much as I did). For coders, we use the 'do unto others as you would have them do to you' approach, that is, we submit the changes we are recommending along with current coding guidance such as Coding Clinic in advance to either the coding manager or the coder. This provides the coder with the opportunity to review and discuss why she coded it the way she did. Ideally, that discussion can occur face to face between the coder or coding manager and us. —Jane Werner, RHIA, CCS, CRC, AHIMA-approved ICD-10-CM/PCS trainer, vice president of coding compliance, and Bill Remmich, MBA, CCS, COC, AHIMA-approved ICD-10-CM/PCS trainer, FHFMA, assistant vice president of coding compliance.

These comments from "auditors in the trenches" highlight four approaches: face to face, collaborative, educational, and factual.

Presenting the Findings

So, what do you need to do to present your findings? Always re-review your findings prior to meeting with the coder or the physician. No one is infallible, and you may find that you have made a calculation error or overlooked something in the record.

Recognize that adults learn in different ways, so it's best to create a summary document that concisely provides the results in two ways:

- Text
- Pictures (charts, graphs)

There are many people who have very little interest in mathematical information and do not have the time to read a lengthy text-based report. These individuals simply cannot or do not prefer to digest facts in written form. For such people, graphs and charts are an easy, interesting, and quickly absorbable way to understand information in a pictorial form.

For example, in Figure 8.1 there is a chart that displays the coder's performance to his or her peers. It's quickly apparent that the coder needs some additional education on ICD-10-PCS coding but is doing well with ICD-10-CM and achieving the desired diagnosis-related group (DRG). Based on the findings, the auditor should use much of the discussion time to thoroughly review those cases where the ICD-10-PCS coding was incorrect, provide additional reading materials, and show the coder where reference items are in the coding book. It's also important to ask the coder to trace his or her steps in making their code assignment to see whether there may be questions that are being incorrectly responded to in the encoder's path or where there may be opportunities for additional education. Also, you should always ask the coder where he or she believes additional guidance is necessary to achieve a higher score next quarter.

When closing the discussion, the auditor should highlight those areas that the coder did well.

FIGURE 8.1 CODER'S AUDIT RESULTS

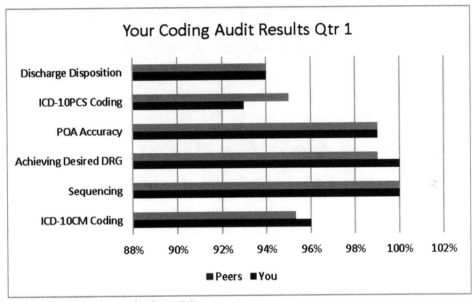

Source: *Rose T. Dunn. Reprinted with permission.*

For physicians, your approach will be similar. Once the audit is completed, the physician's results can be displayed compared to the peers' results in the specialty. See Figure 8.2. This display provides a starting point for the discussion of the audit findings with the physician. Physicians always appreciate having comparative information and are proficient at analyzing data.

FIGURE 8.2 PHYSICIAN X'S CODING AUDIT RESULTS, FIRST QUARTER, 2018

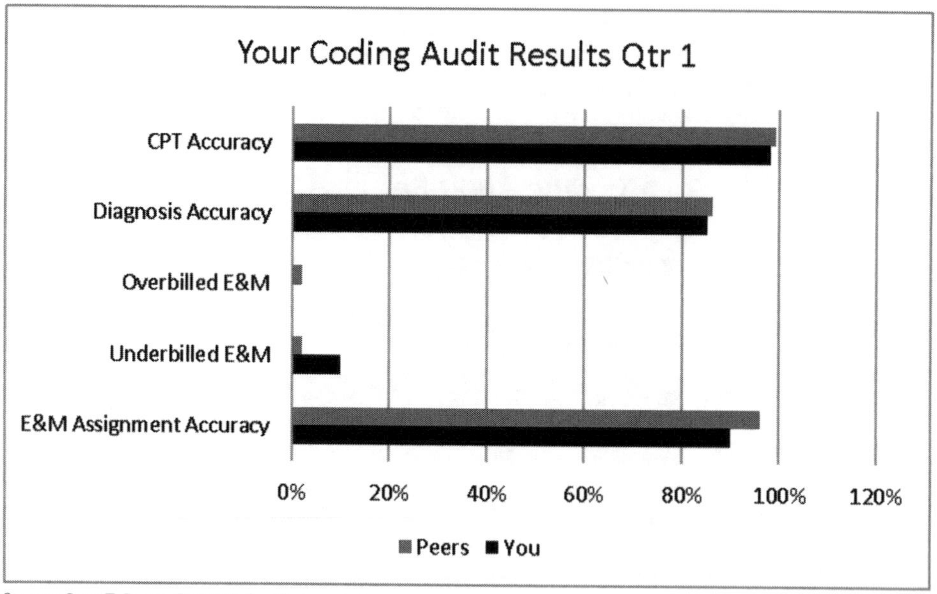

Your Coding Audit Results Qtr 1

CPT Accuracy	
Diagnosis Accuracy	
Overbilled E&M	
Underbilled E&M	
E&M Assignment Accuracy	

0%   20%   40%   60%   80%   100%   120%

■ Peers   ■ You

Source: Rose T. Dunn. Reprinted with permission.

When multiple quarters of data are available, providing the physician with a chart that depicts his or her audit results trended over time can be beneficial. Consider the different formats available for you to display the data that will most effectively communicate the results.

FIGURE 8.3 PHYSICIAN X'S CODING AUDIT RESULTS, FIRST QUARTER, 2017, TO FIRST QUARTER, 2018, DISPLAY OPTIONS

Option 1

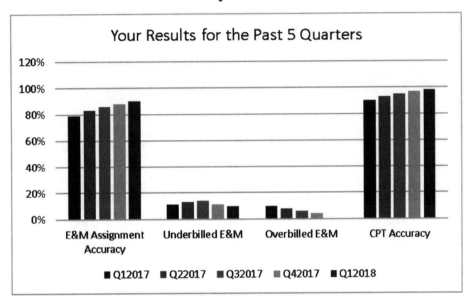

Option 2

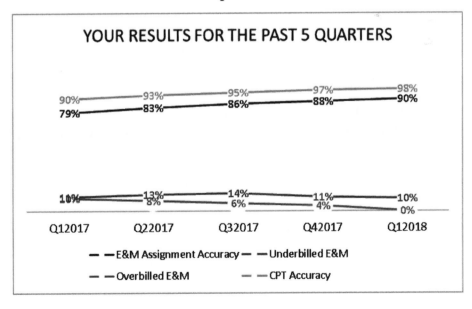

FIGURE 8.3 PHYSICIAN X'S CODING AUDIT RESULTS, FIRST QUARTER, 2017 TO FIRST QUARTER, 2018, DISPLAY OPTIONS (CONT.)

Option 3

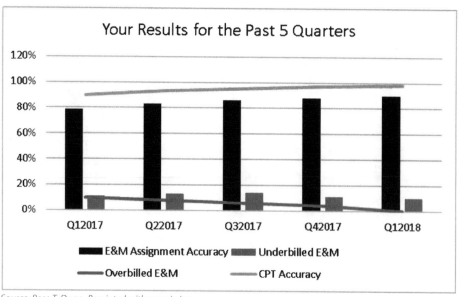

Source: Rose T. Dunn. Reprinted with permission.

Any of the above-given options display the progress made by the physician. Options two and three require the physician to compare the legend to the results, while option one displays the legend directly below the results. Be sure to use colors discriminately. Also, remember that some readers may be colorblind. This may require using black hash or dotted bars and lines for the graphs. In this case, combo graphs such as option three may be a better approach, whereby you can use solid and dotted bars and solid and hashed lines.

FIGURE 8.4 PHYSICIAN X'S CODING AUDIT RESULTS, WITH HASH LINES IN GRAY/BLACK

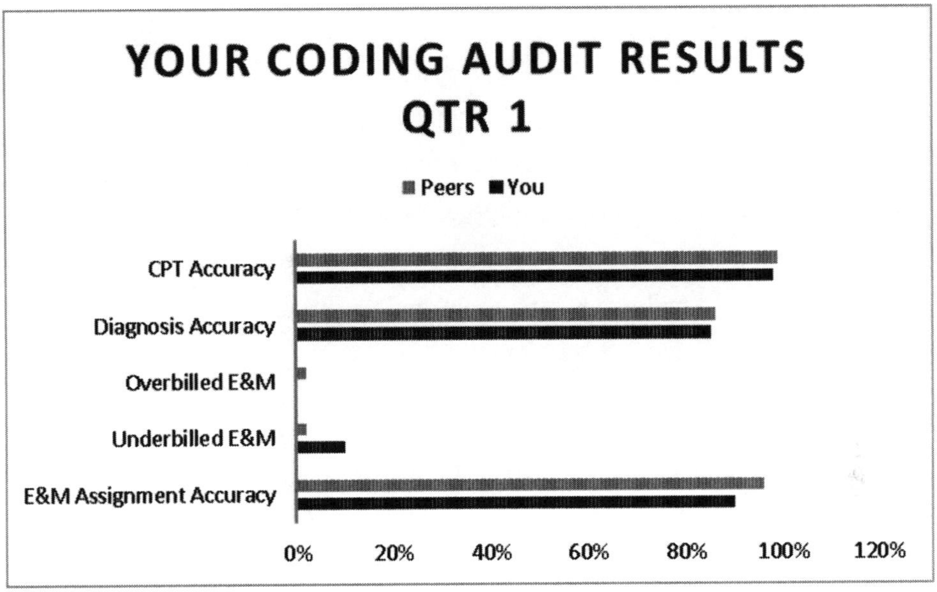

Source: Rose T. Dunn. Reprinted with permission.

Finally, on an annual basis, you may wish to provide physicians and other billing providers with the physician's bell curve of total encounters for the year compared with the CMS data for the same specialty.

To do the comparison, first collect the frequency data for the specialty from the CMS data (see Chapter 7). Enter that data into a spreadsheet by E/M level. Then pull a frequency report from your billing system for the physician. Calculate the total encounters by E/M level and enter into the spreadsheet. From this data you can create the bell curve chart for the provider compared to CMS. When audits are done for several providers of the same specialty, then it is beneficial to display physician A's bell curve beside the total group's bell curve.

Looking at the Documentation

Frese shares that "it is very helpful to look at the provider's actual clinical documentation with the provider during the feedback session. Use it to illustrate points, both positive and negative, and provide recommendations during the discussion of the cases. All in all, to be successful with attempts to change or reinforce behavior with documentation and coding, establishing a respectful relationship and willingness to "listen" and work together are essential for success."

To achieve what Frese is saying requires preparation on your part. Ensuring you are up to date on the latest coding or documentation rules pertaining to the provider's specialty is critical. Also, as discussed earlier, refreshing yourself on your findings in advance of meeting with a coder or provider is essential. You can tag certain cases to emphasize points you wish to make with the provider and print out certain pages of the record to allow you to highlight certain comments in the progress notes, history and physical, or other documents.

Follow Up

Based on your discussion with the coder or provider, changes may need to be made to your final report. Promptly submit your revised final report to the coder (or coding manager) and the provider. After a few days have passed, ensure the revised report was received and ask whether there are any follow-up questions. Enter any data necessary into your trending reports so it is available for the next time. Some additional tips for communicating with physicians appear in the downloadable appendix of this book.

Closing the loop on your audit activities with providers and coders necessitates reviewing the results with them. These individuals may be anxious about the results, so using a collaborative, educational approach can relieve some of the stress for both you and the individual audited. Face-to-face sessions are ideal to be able to gauge whether the individual understands the findings and guidance you have shared as well as to gain their perspectives. Face-to-face sessions also allow you to look at the cases together and understand how the provider or coder translated the documentation into the code(s) assigned. Providing authoritative resources and reference materials that the individual can refer to in the future is beneficial and can help you explain some of the changes you recommended.

Closing Thoughts

In this book, we have discussed why audits are important, how to structure an audit, why prioritizing topics is important, the value of creating an audit schedule, selecting a sample, and presenting your findings. In today's environment, the external scrutiny is tremendous, and our chapter on payer audits explains why. But are there other activities that coding compliance auditors can lead? We discussed the auditor's role in denial management and how taking the lead on coding education fits into the coding compliance auditor's job description.

Leading the education initiative

The coding compliance auditor must keep on top of changing coding rules, new codes, and new clinical services, procedures, and techniques that may impact the choice of codes. The auditor should establish a coding education schedule that includes:

1. Review of *Coding Clinic* quarterly reports. These reports include new guidance that directly apply to appropriate coding for reporting and billing purposes. Review the contents of each with the coding team and issue a short quiz to confirm comprehension of the report's content.

2. Examine the ICD-10-CM, ICD-10-PCS, and CPT-4® code changes. These changes occur annually. The ICD-10 codes are updated annually on October 1, and CPT and HCPCS codes are updated annually on January 1. All code set updates are announced in the *Federal Register* several months prior to their effective date. The coding auditor can start reviewing the changes and prepare educational handouts or PowerPoint slides for the coding team.

3. Attending grand rounds. Attending the grand rounds, which often occurs at teaching facilities with attending and resident physicians, has two advantages. First, this is a forum where new clinical techniques and procedures are discussed and where new technologies are reviewed. During these discussions, physicians can be identified who may be willing to speak directly to the coding team about complex new procedures. Second, it is an ideal forum to share coding and documentation tidbits and interact with the clinical team while advocating for the coding team.

4. Sharing Cooperating Parties discussions. The Cooperating Parties meet throughout the year. Their discussions are open and available through WebEx. At these sessions, new codes and new coding rules are discussed. Listening to these sessions provides the coding auditor with a heads-up on new coding developments that can be shared with the coding team.

Monitoring the regulatory environment

We discussed the vital role that the coding compliance auditor plays in denial management. The auditor is also encouraged to monitor the topics that are on the OIG's priority list and the focus topics of the Recovery Audit Contractors. However, the auditor can demonstrate his or her value in other ways by staying on top of other external auditor initiatives and managing the audit process when an external audit occurs.

In addition to audits we discussed in earlier chapters, the Health Effectiveness Data and Information Set (HEDIS) audits are conducted by approximately 90% of health plans. There are no overpayment demands with these audits, but they could impact the provider's profile. Understanding the HEDIS criteria and coaching the physician practices on these elements throughout the year may enhance the provider's profile.

Audits by upper-level governmental agencies such as the Safeguard Services, Zone Program Integrity Contractor, and the Affirmative Civil Enforcement all have more severe consequences, including involving the Department of Justice and the OIG and pursuing criminal and civil prosecution for fraudulent practices. Should one of these audits occur at the facility, the coding compliance auditor along with the billing charge auditor should prepare complete records and validate that all charges are properly ordered and documented, and all codes are validated based on the clinical documentation in the record.

When making copies, Jacqueline Thelian recommends making four copies, one for each of the following: your office, the insurance company, your attorney, and the coding and billing auditors (Thelian, 2017). Additionally, she recommends including any tracings or images for diagnostic test ordered and reported in the record. Knowing the appeal process and stages will make the auditor a go-to resource for all in the organization, including the organization's legal counsel (Thelian, 2017).

There are numerous opportunities for coding compliance auditors to pursue and review in a healthcare organization. Their findings will assist the organization in its revenue integrity pursuits and compliance mission. Serving as an auditor means being a resource for the coding team. The auditor's educational role is inherent in the position. Establishing an education calendar will provide structure to the delivery of educational offerings as well as serve as a motivator for the auditor to dig into new coding rules and remain up to date with clinical developments that could impact how codes are applied for new clinical techniques, procedures, and technologies. Stepping in and managing external audits may allow the auditor to protect the organization from unreasonable refund demands and become a trusted source of information for the organization's leadership and legal counsel.

REFERENCE

Thelian, J. 2017. "When the Auditor Comes Knocking, Will You Be Ready?" BC *Advantage Magazine,* p. 20–22. September/October 2017. Issue 12.5.